GENOMICS AND WORLD HEALTH

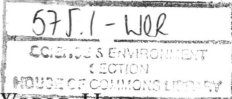
GENOMICS AND WORLD HEALTH

REPORT OF THE ADVISORY COMMITTEE ON

HEALTH RESEARCH

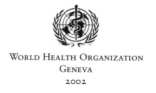
WORLD HEALTH ORGANIZATION
GENEVA
2002

WHO Library Cataloguing-in-Publication Data

World Heath Organization. Advisory Committee on Health Research.

   Genomics and world health / report of the Advisory Committee on Health Research.

   1. Genomics 2. Genome 3. World health 4. Delivery of health care
   5. Developing countries

   ISBN 92 4 154554 2   (NLM Classification: QZ 50)

Typeset and printed in Canada.
Design and production: Digital Design Group, Newton, MA USA

Contents

Acknowledgements

The writing team for this Report was comprised of David Weatherall (Principal/Lead Writer), Dan Brock and Heng-Leng Chee. Members of the WHO Advisory Committee on Health Research (Zulfiqar Bhutta, Barry Bloom, Mahmoud Fathalla-Committee Chair, Marian Jacobs, Gerald Keusch, Maxime Schwartz, Gita Sen, Fumimaro Takaku, Cesar Victora, Lars Walloe, Judith Whitworth) provided extensive comments and inputs to various drafts of the Report prepared by the writing team. David Carr provided invaluable editorial support throughout the preparation of the Report. Williamina Wilson provided expert editorial assistance on the final draft of the Report. Tikki Pang coordinated the process for preparation and development of the Report and the Department of Research Policy & Cooperation, WHO, Geneva, Switzerland acted as secretariat. Invaluable secretarial assistance was provided throughout by Liz Rose and Daniéle Doebeli. Important inputs were also received from a large number of individuals who participated in the various consultations and from WHO staff members (listed in Annexes B2 and B3). Additional material, advice and assistance on various aspects of the Report and its preparation were provided by Bob Cook-Deegan, Jo Cooper, Sigurdur Gudmundsson, Eva Harris, Juntra Karbwang, Victor McKusick, Alex Mauron, Richard Moxon, Chris Newbold, Tim Peto, Abha Saxena, Manju Sharma, Sacha Sidjanski, John Sulston and Andrew Simpson. William R. Brinkley was responsible for the cover design and Marc Kaufman for lay-out design and production.

FOREWORD FROM THE DIRECTOR GENERAL

The announcement of the sequencing of the human genome in 2001 represents an unprecedented milestone in the advancement of our knowledge on the molecular basis of life itself. Together with the advances made in the deciphering of the genomes of many disease-causing microorganisms and their vectors, it is clear that the science of genomics holds tremendous potential for improving health globally.

The information generated by genomics will, over time, provide major benefits for the prevention, diagnosis and management of communicable and genetic diseases as well as other common killers or causes of chronic ill health including cardiovascular diseases, cancer, diabetes, and mental illnesses. It is thus timely and appropriate for WHO to examine the implications of advances in genomics and other critical areas of biotechnology. For this reason, I have asked the Advisory Committee on Health Research (ACHR) to prepare this Report.

The Report focuses on the expectations, concerns and possibilities for the use of new genomic knowledge in improving world health. The specific challenge is how we can harness this knowledge and have it contribute to health equity, especially among developing nations. It is a reality that most genomic and biotechnology research is presently carried out in the industrialized world, and is primarily market-driven. Genomics also needs to be applied to the health problems of the developing world. It is crucial that we actively seek means to involve developing country scientists in innovative biotechnology.

The present Report points out that the genomics revolution has brought with it many complex scientific, economic, social and ethical concerns. These need to be carefully addressed, debated and considered. Recent developments in cloning and stem cell therapy, for example, have raised serious ethical, moral and safety concerns. It follows that societies also need to be better prepared for the era of genomics and its consequences. Public education, understanding and trust on the key issues in genomics is a basic pre-requisite. It is also vital that genomics be considered in the wider context of health and that a relevant balance is maintained in research, development and health care provision between the more conventional and well-tried approaches of clinical research, epidemiology and public health and work directed at the medical applications of genomics, both in the context of individual countries and globally.

Strong international leadership is required to achieve these laudable aims. WHO is committed to facilitating this by promoting international partnerships and cooperation strategies to ensure that the fruits of the genomics revolution are equitably shared by all.

Gro Harlem Brundtland, MD, MPH,
Director-General of WHO,
Geneva, Switzerland.

Executive Summary

Introduction

1. The objective of WHO is the attainment by all peoples of the highest possible level of health. This Report, prepared under the auspices of the Advisory Committee on Health Research (ACHR), is addressed primarily to the 191 WHO Member States, the global and six regional secretariats of WHO, and WHO representatives stationed in 110 countries. It is intended to highlight the relevance of genomics for health care worldwide, with a particular focus on its potential for improving health in developing countries. The stimulus for the Report came from the announcement of the sequencing of the human genome, and the great public interest that this has engendered. Concomitant with the success of the human genome project, the genomes of a number of important pathogens, disease vectors and plants are being characterized; it may be that the knowledge that this work generates will, in the short term, provide greater health gains for the populations of developing countries.

2. This Report should be considered in the context of the primacy of fundamental overarching strategies to improve health, for example through alleviation of poverty, development of health systems, improved education and classical public health approaches to disease control and prevention and health promotion. All Member States must ensure that genome technology is used to reduce rather than exacerbate global inequalities in health status.

Background

3. The application of knowledge gained from the characterization of the genomes of several organisms, including the human genome, holds considerable potential for the development of new health care innovations over the coming decades. It is clear, however, that this new field presents a series of highly complex scientific, economic, social and ethical issues.

4. In order to inform WHO strategy in this crucial area, the Director-General of WHO requested in January 2001 that the ACHR prepare a Report on the likely impact of the genomics revolution on world health, with a primary focus on the implications for developing countries. In order to gather the inputs of key stakeholder groups, three international consultative meetings were held in June and July 2001 in Geneva, Switzerland, Brasilia, Brazil and Bangkok, Thailand. This Report builds upon the evidence presented and consensus points reached at these consultations and was enhanced greatly by discussions with, and feedback from, WHO staff members.

THE SCIENTIFIC BASIS FOR A POTENTIAL REVOLUTION IN HEALTH CARE

5. The characteristics of all living organisms reflect the complex interactions between their genetic make-up, their environment, and the long history of the milieu in which they are raised. It is now recognized that many of the biological functions which result from this interplay will ultimately be explained in terms of biochemical mechanisms which, in turn, reflect the activities of the genes which regulate them. Hence, in recent years there has been a growing emphasis in medical research on the analysis of disease mechanisms at the level of molecules and cells in general, and genes in particular.

6. The sum total of genetic information of an individual, which is encoded in the structure of deoxyribonucleic acid (DNA), is called a genome. The study of the genome is termed "genomics." Recently, the order of most of the chemical building blocks, or bases, which constitute the DNA of the genomes of human beings (estimated to amount to three billion), several other animal species, and a variety of human pathogens and plants has been determined. Over the next few years this remarkable achievement will be completed and augmented by research into functional genomics, which aims to characterize the many different genes that constitute these genomes and their variability of action. Such research will also determine how these genes are regulated and interact with each other and with the environment to control the complex biochemical functions of living organisms, both in health and disease.

7. Work in the field of genomics will also offer completely new insights into the mechanisms of human and animal development and ageing;

and, because our evolutionary history is written in our DNA, it will start to unravel our genetic roots and help us to understand the relationships between and within different species.

THE POTENTIAL OF GENOMICS FOR HEALTH CARE

8. It is now believed that the information generated by genomics will, in the long-term, have major benefits for the prevention, diagnosis and management of many diseases which hitherto have been difficult or impossible to control. These include communicable and genetic diseases, together with other common killers or causes of chronic ill-health, including cardiovascular disease, cancer, diabetes, the major psychoses, dementia, rheumatic disease, asthma, and many others.

9. Research directed at pathogen genomes will enhance our understanding of disease transmission and of virulence mechanisms and how infective agents avoid host defences, information which should enable the development of new classes of diagnostics, vaccines and therapeutic agents. Taken together with the knowledge generated from the characterization of the genomes of vectors that transmit infectious diseases, and of the human genome, the field of genomics may also lead to new approaches for vector control and begin to reveal why there are such wide individual variations in susceptibility to these conditions in human populations.

10. Except for genetic diseases that result from a single defective gene, most common diseases result from environmental factors, together with variations in individual susceptibility, which reflect the action of several genes. Many forms of cancer appear to result from acquired damage to specific sets of genes, oncogenes, usually due to exposure to environmental agents. It is likely that further research into disease-susceptibility genes will help us to understand the mechanisms of these diseases and enable more focused approaches to their prevention and treatment. In particular, it should lead to the discovery of specific molecular targets for therapy, provide information that will allow treatment to be tailored to individual needs, and, in the longer-term, generate a new approach to preventive medicine based on genetic susceptibility to environmental hazards.

11. Some of the claims for the medical benefits of genomics have undoubtedly been exaggerated, particularly with respect to the time-scales required for them to come to fruition. Because of these uncertainties, it is vital that genomics research is not pursued to the detriment of the well-established methods of clinical practice, and clinical and epidemiological research. Indeed, for its full exploitation it will need to be integrated into clinical research involving patients and into epidemiological studies in the community. It is crucially important that a balance is maintained in medical practice and research between genomics and these more conventional and well-tried approaches.

12. Although this Report focuses on human and pathogen genomics, the consequences of research into plant genomics and the genetic modification of crops has great potential for improving human health through nutritional gains and the production and delivery of vaccines and therapeutic agents.

TECHNOLOGICAL RISKS AND ETHICAL, SOCIAL AND ECONOMIC IMPLICATIONS OF GENOMICS

13. Because many of the medical benefits of genomics research may, at least at first, be very expensive, there is a danger that these new developments will increase the disparity in health care within and between countries. There are particular concerns that inequalities in health care will be accentuated by the current trends in the management of intellectual property, particularly the patenting of basic genomic information.

14. The lack of biotechnology and information technology development in many developing countries is also of concern. While there are major international research programmes focused on HIV/AIDS, tuberculosis and malaria, the control of many important infections will undoubtedly fall to individual countries or regions. The lack of market incentives for the global pharmaceutical industry to pursue genomics-based research and development towards neglected diseases of the world's poor countries means that, unless their biotechnology capacity is developed or mechanisms can be fostered to facili-

tate greater investment from public and private institutions in both developed and developing countries, the potential of genomics to combat these diseases will be not be realized and existing inequalities in health will be exacerbated.

15. In genomics research and its medical application, familiar ethical issues such as informed consent, confidentiality, and avoiding discrimination and stigmatization take on different forms because of both the nature of genetic information and the specific social and economic contexts of individual countries. These questions need to be debated widely so that countries can establish their own ethical framework and regulatory structures based on principles which have been agreed internationally.

16. There are many aspects of recombinant DNA technology, particularly those which involve the manipulation of human or animal genomes, which require regulation on matters of public safety, the health of research workers, risks to the environment and the potential for social and political misuse. In addition, the use of genetically modified plants will necessitate the development of more effective mechanisms to minimize the risks to consumers, and to biodiversity and the rights of traditional farmers. In many countries, particularly those which are introducing recombinant DNA technology for the first time, adequate regulatory frameworks do not exist to safeguard against these risks and hazards. The establishment of these structures represents a crucial priority.

17. Societies need to be better prepared for the era of genomics and its consequences. Genomics research is complex and an understanding of its medical potential and the ethical issues involved requires a basic understanding of the principles of genetics. This will only be achieved by a major effort to increase the quality of education in this field at all levels, with particular emphasis on improving science teaching and the introduction of the principles of ethics to schoolchildren. The development of mechanisms to communicate these concepts effectively and engage the general public in an informed dialogue regarding these issues is equally important.

RECOMMENDATIONS

18. The following recommendations are set against a background of current and anticipated future requirements of WHO Member States. Member States will need to make their own assessments of these requirements and their relative priorities. Member States should, with the encouragement of WHO, explore opportunities for regional collaboration, collaboration between developed and developing countries and between developing countries. To support its Member States, WHO will need to:
   ■ enhance its capacity for responding to requests for technical cooperation from Member States;
   ■ exercise its normative function for setting standards and guidelines and harmonization of procedures;
   ■ fulfil its advocacy role to ensure that the benefits of these scientific advances are shared by all countries, rich or poor.

Technical cooperation between WHO and its Member States
19. Given the remarkable speed of progress in genomics research, the coming decades are likely to see an enormous expansion of this field, with important potential for its clinical application to benefit health care globally. Member States need to be prepared for this completely new approach to medical research and practice. Furthermore, the capacity for genomics research and downstream biotechnology research and development varies enormously between countries, and, if uncorrected, this situation will undoubtedly exacerbate existing inequalities in health. Member States should consider undertaking analyses of their existing biotechnological capacity as a basis upon which to develop their strategic priorities in this field.

To assist its Member States, WHO should develop the capacity to evaluate advances in genomics, to anticipate their potential for research and clinical application in the many different environments of the Member States and to assess their effectiveness and cost in comparison with current practice. Where appropriate, WHO may respond to requests from Member States to enhance their capacity in this research field.

20. Easily transferable and well-tried clinical applications of DNA technology exist which could provide immediate benefits for health care in many countries, the control of the common inherited disorders of haemoglobin being one example. This would enable these countries to develop capabilities in other crucial research fields, such as the genetic epidemiology of communicable and non-communicable diseases.

Through building on and expanding its existing capacity in human genetics, WHO could provide technical assistance to Member States to aid them in establishing centres for clinical genetics and genetic research programmes targeted to their particular health problems — facilitating the transfer of appropriate technologies through regional meetings, the establishment training programmes based on collaboration between developed and developing countries and the continued development of regional networking. In addition, WHO could assist Member States in establishing public education and genetic counselling programmes, which are an essential precursor to technology transfer of this type.

21. An important priority for many developing Member States will be to utilize the technologies of pathogen and human genomics for the control and management of communicable diseases. Universities, public research institutions and the commercial sector will all be key participants in research and development programmes to generate new health care products in line with local priorities. Capacity building to enable such programmes might be achieved most effectively through the development of academic, public research and industrial partnerships between developed and developing countries and between developing countries themselves, encouraged by tax or other incentives, and through extensive networking within regions where there is evolving expertise in biotechnology.

The convening power of WHO may be used to facilitate the establishment of such partnerships.

22. In order to participate in genomics research and utilize the vast quantities of genomic data that are being generated, much of which is being released freely into the public domain, Member States must

develop a critical mass of expertise in bioinformatics. There is already a shortage of trained scientists and technicians in this crucially important discipline, even in developed countries. As a first step, countries may decide to examine their current capacity in bioinformatics and identify existing shortfalls.

WHO could provide technical assistance to Member States in developing their bioinformatics capabilities by facilitating regional networking, collaboration between developed and developing countries, and the development of short-term training programmes. WHO may build on its existing activities in this field.

23. All Member States will need to evolve appropriate national frameworks to consider the ethical implications of genomics research and its applications in their own unique social, cultural, economic and religious context. Furthermore, in many countries, there is currently a critical shortage of personnel trained in bioethics to contribute to the analysis of these issues.

WHO could play an important role in working with Member States to assist them in establishing ethical review structures, disseminating the major principles on which programmes of bioethics suited to local needs should evolve, and supporting international and regional training programmes in bioethics.

WHO normative function

24. It is important that the perspectives of all Member States are represented in international debates regarding the ethical implications of advances in genomics.

WHO is in a position to adopt a crucial leadership role in bioethics, particularly as it relates to genomics and world health. Such an activity could be focused through the new Ethics in Health Initiative and build on the work undertaken by WHO ELSI (ethical, legal and social implications) of Genomics Programme over the last two years. Through these mechanisms and working in close collaboration with other organizations with activities in this area, WHO should be ideally placed to anticipate new ethical issues and to provide well-informed advice and leadership.

25. Because this field is evolving a new and completely unexplored technology, it is vital that Member States develop appropriate regulatory structures to monitor and control the commercial and medical applications of genomics research.

WHO could play a major role in providing advice and assistance to the governments of Member States about how best to establish simple regulatory systems for the wide variety of technologies that are being developed from genomics.

An advocacy role for WHO

26. Because genomics is a new and rapidly developing field, there remain many uncertainties about the validity of the current predictions for the benefits to health which will accrue from this endeavor, and even greater concerns about the time-scale involved.

It is vital that WHO advocates the maintenance of a relevant balance in research, development and health care provision between the more conventional and well-tried approaches of clinical research, epidemiology and public health and work directed at the medical applications of genomics, both in the context of individual Member States and globally.

27. There are profound concerns that current practices in intellectual property, particularly regarding the granting of patents on fundamental genomic information, will place many Member States at a considerable disadvantage in realizing equitably the health care potential of genomics.

WHO should adopt a proactive role as an advocate for health equity in international debates on intellectual property issues.

28. It should be more widely recognized that the health problems of the developing world, including both communicable and non-communicable diseases, are *global* concerns. Furthermore, diseases which have hitherto been localized to these countries will increasingly impact developed countries. There is a critical need for greater investment at a global level in research directed at the health prob-

lems of developing countries, including research to utilize the potential of genomics.

There is a clear role for WHO in advocating an increase in the availability of resources for genomics research targeted to the health needs of developing countries.

29. In all Member States, there is a crucial need to improve awareness and understanding of genetics in general, and of the medical potential of genomics in particular, not just among the general public, but also among governments, health services administrators, and the medical profession itself. If this is not achieved it will be impossible for society to enter into an informed debate about the ethical issues involved, and there is a danger that those who administer health services will be unable to distinguish between hyperbole and reality in a new and rapidly expanding research field.

WHO advocacy will be important in improving knowledge of this field at every level — in schools, among the public, in medical education, in health care administration, and in government. WHO could also provide technical assistance and advice to Member States in establishing educational and public engagement programmes.

CONCLUSION

30. In summary, WHO should ensure that the proven benefits from this field for the prevention and management of disease are made available, as they emerge, to the developing countries. At the same time, WHO should provide technical assistance and normative guidance and, where appropriate, adopt a strong advocacy role to enable its Member States to develop the scientific, biotechnological, regulatory and ethical bases on which future advances can be applied to improve the health of their populations.

1. INTRODUCTION

The announcement in June 2000 of the partial completion of the Human Genome Project, and the publication of this remarkable achievement in February 2001, was accompanied by the widely stated prediction that it would lead to a revolution in medical research and patient care. Hence, in January 2001 the Director-General of WHO requested that the Advisory Committee on Health Research (ACHR) prepare a Report on the likely impact of genomics on global health, with a particular focus on the implications for developing countries.

The objective of WHO is the attainment of the highest possible level of health by all the peoples of the world. Therefore, the role of genomics for medical practice has had to be considered in the context of strategies to improve the health of populations which are still suffering from the effects of poverty, a lack of basic health systems and a high prevalence of infectious disease, those which are facing the increasing health burden of an ageing population and the intractable diseases of middle and old age, and others which are passing through the demographic and epidemiological transitions between these extremes. Furthermore, it was important for the Report to examine the potential risk that genome technology might exacerbate global health inequalities, and to consider the complex ethical issues which might arise from this new field in the context of the different religious and cultural values of the individual Member States of WHO.

Although the impetus for the Report came from the announcement of the partial completion of the Human Genome Project, the ideas that underlie the potential of this new field for improvements in health care first started to be aired in the middle of the 20th century. Since this time, there has been an increasing emphasis in medical research directed at the analysis of disease mechanisms at the level of cells and molecules. This evolution towards what is sometimes called "molecular medicine" has resulted from an appreciation of the importance of genetics in understanding pathology, together with the development of recombinant DNA technology which has made it possible to isolate and characterize genes from a wide range of organisms, including humans.

At first sight it is not obvious why genetics has come to play such a central role in our thinking about disease. After all, although many diseases can be traced through families because they result from a single defective gene, with a few exceptions they are rare and do not amount to a major health burden. On the other hand, most common diseases are the result of infectious agents or other environmental factors, modified to some degree by variations in pathogen virulence or host susceptibility; and for many of these diseases the cause is unknown. However, two major changes in our thinking about the pathogenesis of disease have highlighted the importance of genetics for an understanding of disease mechanisms. First, any disease process, whether it is the virulent properties of a microorganism that enable it to invade tissues or the pre-cancerous changes in the respiratory tract which follow years of exposure to tobacco smoke, can be explained ultimately in biochemical terms which, in turn, reflect gene function. Second, it has become clear that there is a remarkable degree of individual variation in susceptibility to noxious environmental agents and that this is genetically determined; defining and understanding the actions of the genes involved should, therefore, lead to a better understanding of the underlying pathology of disease.

In short, because genes encode the information required for every biological function, a better understanding of how this is achieved is equally germane to the study of disease as it is to an understanding of normal function. It was such thinking that when the tools of molecular genetics started to become available in the 1970's spawned the new fields of molecular pathology and molecular medicine.

It should be emphasized that this new focus on genetics in medical research and practice does not, as is sometimes suggested, reflect the genetic deterministic view which has it that we are completely at the mercy of our genes and have no control over our destinies. We are what we are as the result of a complex interplay between our genetic make-up, our environment and the cultural milieu in which we are raised. Our genes, because they carry the instructions for the complex biochemical processes that underpin all the essential biochemical activities of living organisms, are but one, albeit central, part of this complex interplay.

Over the last 20 years important progress has been made towards an understanding of the molecular basis of many single-gene disorders, that is conditions that follow a simple Mendelian mode of inheritance. Much has also been learnt about the genetic mechanisms of congenital malformation and mental retardation. A start has been made towards a better understanding the genetic component of the major killers or causes of ill health of middle life: heart disease, stroke, diabetes, the major psychoses, and cancer, for example. New technologies have offered insights into individual variability in response to infection, and the protean ways in which infective agents can bypass both the immune system and therapeutic agents. These advances have spawned a major new biotechnology industry. Although progress in translating them into day to day clinical practice has been slow, enough is known already to suggest that molecular genetics will play an increasingly important role in patient care in the future.

Advances in this field are also helping to answer some of the broader questions of human biology. They are playing a central part in elucidating the mechanisms of evolution and are also making some progress towards enhancing our understanding of more complex issues, such as how a fertilized egg develops into a mature adult and the nature of the mechanisms involved in the process of ageing. They are also starting to yield some understanding of the extremely complex interactions between nature and nurture which underlie human behaviour.

The announcement of the success of the Human Genome Project has given an enormous impetus to this new field of biological and medical research. Genetic information is encoded by the structure of deoxyribonucleic acid (DNA). The sum total of this information for any organism is called its *genome*. The study of the genome is termed genomics. Recently, almost the complete sequence of the three billion (3×10^9) chemical building blocks, or bases, of the DNA which constitutes the human genome has been determined. This remarkable achievement will probably be completed within the next two or three years. Genes are lengths of DNA which carry the information to make functional products — most often proteins, or parts of them; some proteins are encoded by more than one gene. It is currently estimated that the human genome contains between 28 000 and 40 000 genes. Although it is already clear that it will take a long time to determine the function of all of them, and how they interact one with another and with the environment, it is believed that the information that will be generated from this complex task will have a profound effect on the provision of health care in the future. But it is equally clear that it will raise new sets of ethical issues which have not been encountered before in clinical practice and which strike at the very heart of the basis of human nature and how far we wish to go in exploiting and modifying our genetic make-up.

Side by side with the Human Genome Project there have been other genome sequencing projects which, at least in the short term, may have even more important implications for global health. Major progress has been made towards sequencing the genomes of a broad range of human pathogens, work which has direct application for the prevention, diagnosis, and management of communicable disease. Similarly, the determination of the genome sequences of a variety of other organisms is well advanced, information which will be invaluable in helping to determine the functions of both the human and pathogen genomes.

It must be emphasized that molecular genetics and the fruits of the genome projects will not replace the well-established patterns of medical practice and research. Good clinical care will still be based on history taking, detailed physical examination, and well-tried laboratory and other ancillary investigations, backed up by evidence-based therapy and good pastoral care. Similarly, medical research will continue to rely heavily on clinical epidemiology, clinical studies of patients and whole-animal physiology. The sophisticated tools of molecular genetics, while they are undoubtedly an extremely valuable new acquisition to this well-tried armamentarium, will have to be integrated into our current approaches to clinical investigation. Indeed, without a unified approach of this kind, in the development of genetic epidemiology for example, it is unlikely that the potential of such tools for the improvement of health care will be realized.

Assessing the likely medical applications of the genome projects and their aftermath is not easy, particularly in relation to the health of those in developing countries. In the excitement generated by the Human Genome Project many medical scientists and the media have claimed that genome technology will provide quick answers to most of our intractable medical problems. This has already caused some disillusionment when these promised advances have not materialized. It is not clear how long it will take for the next stage of the project to evolve, that is to try to determine the function of all our genes and how they interact with one another. It is even less certain how long it will take for the applications of this work to reach the clinic. At the same time the demography of disease is changing rapidly, necessitating a shifting set of priorities for the provision of health care. However, enough is known already about the potential of this new field to provide at least a tentative framework for future action on the part of WHO and its Member States, to whom this Report is addressed.

Due to the fact that genomics research is moving so quickly, and in the light of claims that it will revolutionize health care in the near future, it was important to produce this state-of-the-art Report as quickly as possible. However, in the time available, it was possible to obtain the inputs of many of the Member States and key stakeholder groups at three international consultative meetings held in Geneva, Switzerland, Brasilia, Brazil and Bangkok, Thailand, together with valuable contributions and feedback from WHO staff members. In recognition of the enormous breadth and diversity of this field, and hence the Report's inability to deal with any one aspect in detail, it contains a short bibliography for further reading together with key reference sources for each section (Annex C).

2.   GENOMICS AND THE GENOME PROJECTS

Contents

2.1   INTRODUCTION

Many of the concepts of genomics, though relatively straightforward, may not be familiar to every reader of this Report. The introduction to this Section and the Glossary at the end of the Report are directed at those who are new to this field. Though it is not essential to have a full understanding of the complexities of genomics to appreciate its potential importance for the betterment of human health, it is nevertheless helpful to have some acquaintance with the basic underlying principles.

This Section then goes on to describe how the advent of recombinant DNA technology in the 1970s revolutionized our ability to characterize the genetic basis of disease and how the Human Genome Project was essentially a natural progression of this work. It provides an introduction to the powerful tools of functional genomics, which are allowing researchers to begin to understand the complex mechanisms through which genes and their products interact to effect biological function and influence disease processes. Finally, it describes how work to characterize the genomes of pathogens and other organisms will be crucial in realizing the potential of this field to improve human health.

2.2   WHAT ARE GENES AND HOW DO THEY FUNCTION?

With the exception of viruses, which are intracellular parasites, living organisms are divided into two general classes. First, there are eukaryotes whose cells have a complex compartmentalized internal structure; they comprise algae, fungi, plants and animals. Second, there are prokaryotes, single-celled microorganisms with a simple internal organization, which

comprise bacteria and related organisms. Genetic information is transferred from one generation to the next by subcellular structures called
chromosomes. Prokaryotes usually have a single circular chromosome,
while most eukaryotes have more than two and in some cases up to several hundred. For example, in humans there are 23 pairs; one of the pair
is inherited from each parent. Twenty-two pairs are called autosomes and
one pair are called sex chromosomes. The latter are designated X and Y;
females have two X chromosomes (XX) while males have an X and Y
(XY).

A chromosome consists of a tightly packaged length of deoxyribonucleic acid (DNA), together with the proteins that help to define its structure and level of activity. DNA consists of two long strings of nucleotide
bases wrapped round each other. There are four bases: adenine (A), guanine (G), cytosine (C) and thymine (T) (Figure 2.1). Genes are specific
lengths of DNA that encode the information to make a protein or ribonucleic acid (RNA) product. Proteins are remarkably variable in their structure, ranging from the tough collagen that forms connective tissue and
bone, through the fluid haemoglobin that transports oxygen, to thousands
of enzymes, hormones and other biological effectors and their receptors
that drive our body chemistry. Each protein is made up of one or more
chains of amino acids (peptide chains), of which only 20 occur in living
organisms. The different structures and functions of proteins depend on
the order of the amino acids in the peptide chains from which they are
constructed. This is, in turn, determined by the order of nucleotide bases
in the genes which are responsible for their production.

DNA has the remarkable property of self-replication. As cells divide,
so do chromosomes, and each of the pair of DNA strands comes apart and
acts as a template for the synthesis of a new strand. Because of the strict
rules of the pairing of bases (A always pairs with T and C with G), the
new pairs of DNA strands are therefore identical to those from which they
were synthesized. But they are not always quite identical; sometimes mistakes, or mutations, occur. These usually result from the substitution of a
different base; rarely they may involve more extensive structural changes
to genes. While many mutations are neutral, that is they have no effect on
the function of a gene, very occasionally they may alter its properties in a
favourable way, conferring resistance to disease or other environmental
hazards for example. This is the basis for the gradual change in species
during millions of years of evolution. On the other hand, mutations may

Figure 2.1   THE STRUCTURE OF DNA

The diagram on the right is a model of the Watson Crick DNA double helix. The two bands represent the sugar phosphate backbones of the two strands, which run in opposite directions. The vertical line represents the central axis around which the strands wind. The position of the four nucleotide bases, C (cytosine), A (adenine), T (thymine) and G (guanine), is shown, together with the hydrogen bonds (black dots) which link them together. The diagram on the left represents the structure of part of a DNA chain and shows the chain-linked sugar, deoxyribose, and phosphate residues which form the sugar phosphate backbone.

(From Weatherall, 1991 with permission.)

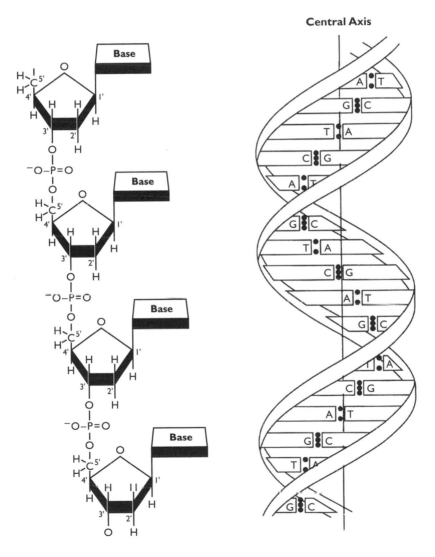

also result in defective gene function and hence lead to disease, or susceptibility to disease.

The relationship between the sequence of nucleotide bases in a gene
and the amino acid composition of a protein is called the genetic code. It
is a triplet, non-overlapping code, such that sets of three bases, called
codons, encode for particular amino acids. When a gene is activated (transcribed) one of its strands of DNA is copied into a mirror-image (or complementary) molecule called messenger ribonucleic acid (mRNA), which
moves from the nucleus to the cytoplasm of a cell, where it acts as a template on which the strings of amino acids are synthesized in the appropriate order, as directed by the codons of the mRNA (Figure 2.2). Some
newly synthesized proteins undergo a process called post-translational
modification during which their structures are changed to convert them to
their functional form.

At first it was thought that there was a direct relationship between all
the sequence of nucleotide bases in a gene and the amino acid sequence of
its protein product. However, things turned out to be more complicated.
Nearly all eukaryotic genes consist of coding regions, called exons, interspersed with non-coding regions called introns. It is still not clear why
genes are split up in this way or exactly what role the introns play.
However, this additional level of complexity means that when the mRNA
precursor is copied from its parent gene, it has to undergo a considerable
amount of processing before it is ready to act as the template for protein
synthesis (Figure 2.2). In particular, the intron sequences have to be
removed and the exon sequences joined together (or spliced) and a certain
amount of chemical modification of both ends of the molecule has to
occur before it is ready to move from the nucleus into the cytoplasm.
Through the development of alternative splicing mechanisms it is possible
for several gene products (proteins) to be encoded by one gene. Since their
genes do not contain introns, things are less complicated in prokaryotes.

A gene is not simply a length of DNA that directs the order of a particular string of amino acids. It must encode appropriate start and stop
signals for protein production. It must also contain regulatory sequences
so that it can be activated at the appropriate time in the correct tissues and
coordinate its activities with those of other genes. Some genes are loosely
regulated and are active in most cells, while others require much tighter
control with regard to the quantity of their product, the tissue in which
they are active, and the period during development in which they are functional.

Figure 2.2   FROM GENE TO PROTEIN

The gene is represented at the top of the figure and consists of shaded regions, exons, separated by unshaded regions, intervening sequences (IVS, introns). The sequences in the flanking regions are key regulatory regions called promoters which are found in all mammalian genes. At each end of the gene there is a non-coding (NC) region. When the gene is transcribed one of the DNA strands is copied into a mirror image messenger RNA (mRNA) precursor. This is processed while in the nucleus such that the intron sequences are removed and the exons joined together and a string of A residues is attached which probably stabilizes the processed mRNA. The latter then passes into the cytoplasm of the cell where it acts as a template for protein production. Amino acids are brought to the template on molecules called transfer RNAs, each of which has three bases which find the appropriate code words (triplets of bases, for their particular amino acid). The mRNA template is read from left to right and the growing peptide chain, incoming transfer RNA and other factors are held in the appropriate configuration to the mRNA on bodies called ribosomes. When the termination codon (e.g.UAA) is reached the ribosomes fall off the mRNA and the finished chain of amino acids is released into the cytoplasm.

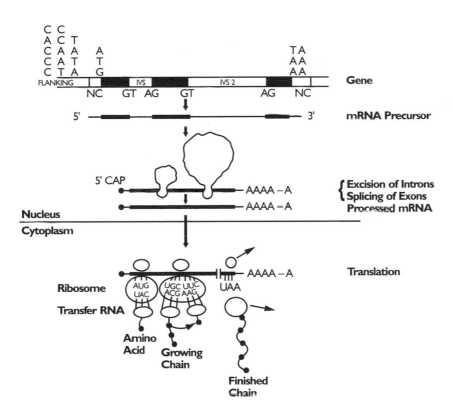

2.3   THE DEVELOPMENT OF MOLECULAR GENETICS

2.3.1   *Classical genetics*

The successes of modern molecular genetics are based firmly on classical genetics which evolved after the rediscovery of the work of Mendel at the beginning of the 20th Century. We have already seen how chromosomes in humans and many other eukaryotic organisms exist in homologous pairs. It follows that their constituent genes must also be present in pairs. We have also seen how the structure of a gene may change as a result of mutation. Hence individual genes may exist in alternate forms, called alleles, only two of which can be present in one individual. Some individuals carry two different allelic forms of a particular gene and are described as heterozygotes for that gene; others have two identical alleles and are called homozygotes. Alleles are said to be dominant if they manifest their phenotypic (recognizable) effect in heterozygotes, and recessive if they cause a phenotypic effect only when present in the homozygous state.

Except during the formation of germ cells, that is sperm or ova, cells divide by a process called mitosis which is preceded by the doubling of each pair of chromosomes, hence ensuring that the two daughter cells each acquire a set of chromosomes identical to the parental cell. During the formation of sperm and ova a different type of cell division occurs called meiosis in which homologous pairs of chromosomes segregate, or separate, to give progeny with half the number of chromosomes (Figure 2.3). Fertilization restores cells to their full chromosome complement. Because chromosomes segregate during germ cell formation, it follows that the two allelic members of a single pair of genes pass to different germ cells during reproduction. This is the basis for Mendel's first law of inheritance, which states that each pair of genes, or alleles, segregate.

These beautifully simple principles provide an explanation for the patterns of inheritance of diseases that result from mutations of a single-gene within families (Box 2.1). Depending on whether the particular condition is dominant or recessive, it will pass through families in a predictable manner showing either a Mendelian recessive or dominant pattern of inheritance or, if the particular gene is on an X chromosome, X-linked recessive or dominant inheritance (Figure 2.4).

Mendel's second law of inheritance deals with the more complicated situation involving the inheritance of different gene pairs. It states that different gene pairs assort to germ cells independently of one another, or in short, non-alleles assort. However, there is one exception to this law

Figure 2.3   Mitotic and meiotic cell division

During mitosis the chromosome number is doubled so that when the cell divides each of the daughter cells has the same number of chromosomes as the parental cell. During meiosis (germ cell formation) there is a second division and the resulting germ cells contain only one or other of the parental chromosomes. Since the latter become closely apposed during homologous pairing there is the opportunity for genetic material to be transferred between them, a process called recombination. This is illustrated at the bottom of the figure.

(From Weatherall, 1991 with permission.)

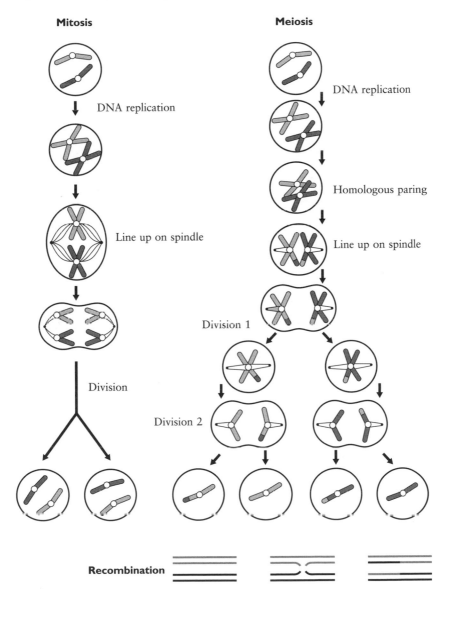

Box 2.1   MENDELIAN INHERITANCE

If a man and a woman have identical genes at the same locus, called **A** for example, they can only produce germ cells (sperm or eggs) of type **A**, and consequently can only have children with a **AA** genotype. If on the other hand, **A** exists in another form (or allele), say and the genotype of the father is **AA** and the mother is **Aa**, then although the father can only produce A germ cells, half the mother's will be **A**, and half will be **a**. The possible genotypes of their children can be worked out as follows.

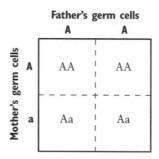

It follows that half the children (shown in the box) will have the genotype **AA**, and half **Aa**. On the other hand, if both parents have the genotype **Aa**, then one quarter of the children will have the genotype **AA**, one quarter the genotype **aa**, and one half the genotype **Aa**, as follows:

Father's germ cells

	A	A
A	AA	Aa
a	Aa	aa

Mother's germ cells

If the **a** allele causes a disease, its appearance in families will depend on whether it is dominantly inherited (expressed in heterozygotes, **Aa**) or recessively inherited (expressed in homozygotes, **aa**). If dominantly inherited, on average half the children of an affected parent will be affected (top figure). If recessively inherited, on average a quarter of the children of **Aa** parents (heterozygotes or carriers) will be affected (**aa**) (bottom figure).

which is absolutely central to an understanding of the medical potential of the Human Genome Project. It is that when two genes are on the same chromosome and particularly if they are located close together, they will tend to be inherited together; the genes are then said to be linked. However, parental chromosomes become closely opposed at meiosis, and crossing over, in the form of reciprocal exchange of the genes between

Figure 2.4   PEDIGREES ILLUSTRATING DIFFERENT FORMS OF
MONOGENIC INHERITANCE

The squares represent males and the circles females. The different generations are represented by Roman numerals and the number of persons in each generation by Arabic numerals. In the family showing autosomal dominant inheritance the open symbols represent normal individuals and the half-shaded symbols affected people. In the two recessive forms of inheritance the open symbols are normal, half shaded are carriers (non-affected) and fully shaded are affected. In X-linked (sex-linked) inheritance, since males only have one X chromosome, they cannot transmit the condition to their sons but all their daughters will be carriers. Female carriers, on average, will have half of their sons affected, depending on which of the X chromosomes is passed down to them; similarly, half their daughters will be carriers.

(From Weatherall, 1991 with permission.)

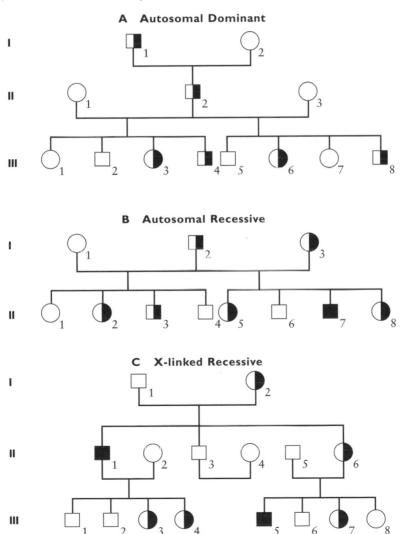

maternal and paternal chromosomes, can occur (Figure 2.3), so that the two characteristics determined by the genes will part in some of the children Such offspring are called recombinants. The closer together a pair of genes are on the same chromosome, the less will be the chance of crossing over. Hence, the number of recombinants in families is a measure of the distance between the genes. The distance separating two loci that show recombination in one out of 100 germ cells is called a map unit, or centimorgan (named after the American geneticist, Thomas Hunt Morgan). Easily identifiable linkage markers now play a central role in enabling us to locate genes involved in disease.

The other major contribution of classical genetics was the recognition of what became known as multifactorial inheritance. It gradually became clear that many characteristics, height and weight for example, do not conform to Mendel's laws of inheritance. The application of statistical methods to analysing this type of inheritance showed that it could be explained by the action of multiple sets of genes, each with a small but additive effect. It is now apparent that many diseases follow this type of inheritance and reflect the interaction of a variety of environmental factors with complex genetic backgrounds of this kind.

Using these concepts a picture emerged of a broad spectrum of genetic disease, both Mendelian and multifactorial, and considerable progress was made towards defining the action of some of the genes involved. However, until it was possible to analyse these genes directly it was impossible to determine how different mutations produce different clinical disorders, and because of the paucity of linkage markers, mapping genomes moved very slowly. This situation changed dramatically in the last quarter of the 20th Century.

2.3.2   Molecular genetics

The revolution in genetics which led to the molecular era was driven by a remarkably sophisticated series of new technologies which evolved in the 1970s (Box 2.2). It became possible to fractionate DNA into pieces of predictable size and insert them into plasmids, small circular entities which are able to divide within bacteria. This process, augmented with the development of more sophisticated vectors of this kind which would accommodate larger pieces of DNA, was used to generate libraries of these recombinant carriers of DNA, which were grown in bacterial cultures. Individual colonies containing genes of interest could then be isolated and grown in sufficient amounts for analysis, a technique which became

Box 2.2   SOME LANDMARKS IN THE APPLICATION OF HUMAN MOLECULAR
GENETICS TO THE STUDY OF DISEASE

Year	Landmark
1941	Genes code for single proteins
1944	Proof that DNA carries genetic information
1949	The concept of sickle cell anaemia as a "molecular disease"
1953	Structure of insulin determined Structure of DNA determined
1956	Monogenic disease due to a single amino acid substitution of the β-chain of haemoglobin
1960	The X-ray crystallographic structure of haemoglobin
1961	The genetic code, messenger RNA, gene regulation
1972	Recombinant DNA, cloning and gene isolation
1974	Direct demonstration of a human gene deletion
1975	Southern blotting*
1976	Proto-oncogenes
1977	DNA sequencing
1978	Human gene library
1979	Restriction fragment length polymorphism used for prenatal diagnosis Stop codon mutation demonstrated in human globin messenger RNA Cellular oncogenes
1979–81	Human genes cloned and sequenced
1985	"Disease genes" isolated by positional cloning Polymerase chain reaction (PCR)
2000	The Human Genome Project — completion of 90% draft

This list shows a few of the milestones in molecular biology and its application to the study of human disease over the second half of the 20ᵗʰ Century. It emphasizes that, by the time that the success of the Human Genome Project was announced, there was a solid base of evidence of the importance of molecular and cell biology for the future of medical practice. From 1980 to 2000, much was learnt about the molecular pathology of monogenic diseases and cancer, and a start was made towards the dissection of the complexities of multifactorial disease.

* *A technique invented by Ed Southern for studying DNA fragments immobilized on nitrocellulose. This method was seminal to advances in human molecular genetics.*

known as cloning, simply because each derivative from individual colonies contained an identical fragment of DNA. Ingenious methods, based on the observation that DNA or RNA will form stable hybrids with partners which are sufficiently similar in base composition, were developed to identify individual genes of interest. Once isolated, a gene could be sequenced, induced to synthesise its products in microorganisms, cultured cells or even in other species, and hence its regulatory regions could be defined.

2.4   CHARACTERIZING THE HUMAN GENOME

2.4.1   The identification of human disease genes

The first human genes to be explored were those for which the gene product was already characterized at the protein level, haemoglobin and the blood clotting factors for example. But in many cases nothing was known about the nature of a particular gene or its product, or the pathological basis for the diseases that resulted from its mutations. Ever since the concept of gene linkage was established it was realized that the way to pinpoint a gene of unknown location and function would be to look for an appropriate inherited marker, a blood group for example, and determine if the unknown gene and the marker stayed together through different generations of a family. If so, the gene that was being sought must be linked to that for the marker. Until the new DNA technology became available there were very few genetic markers with which to carry out linkage studies of this type. However, once the structure of human DNA was analysed it became clear that there is remarkable individual variability and many different families of markers were discovered.

Using DNA linkage markers it was possible to trace genes for diseases through families and determine their approximate location on different chromosomes. It was then possible to "walk" along the chromosome and to isolate the defective gene and, from the order of its bases and a knowledge of the genetic code, to assess the structure of the protein that it would encode, and hence to determine its likely function. This revolutionary procedure, first called reverse genetics and later re-christened positional cloning, led to the discovery of genes for many important monogenic diseases, that is diseases inherited in a Mendelian fashion, and, indeed, has become the principle on which hopes are pinned for studying the genetics of complex multifactorial diseases in the future.

It was from these early successes, and some equally remarkable developments in cancer genetics, that the notion arose that progress in the further exploration of human genetics, both in health and disease, would be greatly advanced if the nucleotide sequence of the entire human genome was determined. In particular, it would lead to the production of much more effective linkage maps and greatly facilitate the identification of genes in regions of the genome that had been identified by linkage analysis or studies which pointed to the association of a disease with a particular linkage marker.

2.4.2   *The Human Genome Project*

When the Human Genome Project was initiated in the mid-1980s the technology for decoding the sequence of DNA, particularly that based on the work of Sanger in Cambridge was still in the early stages of its development. Although it was thought that completely new approaches would be required this did not turn out to be the case. Rather, there was an incremental improvement in the efficiency of the process, largely through the development of automation, robotics and the advent of high-speed machines that moved fragments of DNA through fine capillaries, thus reducing the time taken to carry out sequencing and, equally important, the cost of the procedure. The other major enabling development was the remarkable increase in sophistication of the computer technology used to analyse the vast amount of data that was generated.

The project was carried out independently in the private and public sectors using different though related approaches. One involved a clone-based method which started by cutting up many copies of the genome into small segments which were then inserted into bacterial artificial chromosomes (BACs). These were then inserted into bacteria where they are copied exactly, each time a bacterium divides. This process resulted in clones of identical DNA molecules that could be further analysed and then lined up in order to produce a physical map of the genome. The individual clones were then broken down into small fragments which were re-cloned and the resulting subclones sequenced. The other approach, sometimes nicknamed "shotgun," utilized small-insert clones which were derived directly from genomic DNA rather than from the physical map.

In June 2000, both Celera Genomics, a private company, and the International Human Genome Mapping Consortium, funded by governments and charities in several countries, announced the completion of "working drafts" of the human genome sequence, that is the order of the three billion bases that constitute our genetic make-up (Lander, et al., 2001; Venter et al., 2001). Over the next few years it will be necessary to complete the sequence analysis by closing gaps and resolving various ambiguities. This "finishing" process has already been more or less accomplished for chromosomes 21 and 22 and should be completed for the remainder of the genome by 2003.

2.4.3   Mapping the human genome

As well as the description of its sequence, major progress has been made towards the completion of other forms of analysis of the genome which already have valuable medical applications. While human DNA sequences are 99.9% identical to each other, the remaining 0.1% of variation is of great practical value. In particular, it makes it possible to construct linkage maps, that is to identify DNA markers, rather like towns on a road map.

Progress towards identifying different varieties of DNA markers has been extremely rapid. Coincident with the partial completion of the genome project a map of 1.42 million single nucleotide polymorphisms (SNPs) was published (Sachidanandam et al., 2001). These are sites in the genome at which single nucleotide bases vary from person to person and seem to occur at a frequency of about 1 per 1900 bases. The SNP Map Working Group which carried out this project estimated that it had identified 60 000 SNPs within genes. It is believed that the SNPs will provide valuable markers for linkage or association studies for the study of genetic susceptibility to disease. Because these genetic polymorphisms occur in linked groups, or haplotypes, which differ between individuals, it may be even more valuable to develop a haplotype map for the purpose of gene identification. As well as their potential importance for studying disease associations this extraordinary degree of variability among our genomes offers great possibilities for studying the evolutionary histories of different species.

2.5   FUNCTIONAL GENOMICS

The further understanding of the functions and regulation of the 30 000 or so genes that constitute the human genome will require multidisciplinary research encompassing many different fields.

2.5.1   Annotation of the human genome

The next stage in the human genome project, and one that has to be carried out for the analysis of any genome, is called genome annotation, that is the process of analysing the raw DNA sequence produced by genome sequencing technologies in order to determine its biological significance. This process involves multiple stages, including studies at the levels of the nucleotide sequence itself, the protein products of different genes and, finally, how the different genes and proteins interact with one another and how the whole network is regulated (Baker and Sali, 2001; Stein, 2001).

The process of identifying genes and placing known landmarks into the genome requires a variety of different technologies backed up by sophisticated software algorithms which have been devised to handle gene prediction in different genomes. Using this plethora of tools it is possible, slowly at the moment, to build up a picture of genes, regulatory regions and the extensive areas of repetitive elements which characterize different genomes. However, while this work is continuing, research in the postgenome period is already focusing intensely on the protein products of the human genome.

2.5.2   Proteomics

One of the main ventures in the era of functional genomics will be in what is now termed "proteomics," that is the large-scale analysis of the protein products of genes. The ultimate goal is to try to define the protein complement, or proteome, of cells and how proteins interact with one another. Proteomics is complementary to genomics because it focuses its attention on gene products and hence has enormous potential for medical application (Brenner, 2001).

It is often very difficult to determine the function of proteins from their primary amino acid sequences derived from the DNA sequence of the gene (or genes) which encodes them. In many cases therefore it will be necessary to isolate proteins and to attempt to determine their structures, quantity and location in cells, the various modifications that they undergo, and the way in which they interact with their partners. To achieve these goals a wide range of powerful technologies are being developed. Large-scale facilities are being established for isolating and purifying the protein products of genes which have been expressed in bacteria. The structure of these proteins can then be studied by a variety of different techniques, notably X-ray crystallography and nuclear magnetic resonance (NMR) spectroscopy. The crystallographic analysis of proteins is being greatly facilitated by the use of X-ray beams from a synchrotron radiation source. Crystallography can be facilitated by the introduction of heavy atoms into proteins and it is now becoming possible to introduce this step in bacterial expression systems.

Major advances in automation and data handling are speeding up all these processes. Other approaches, including the application of a technique called the yeast two-hybrid system, are making it possible to identify which protein interacts with which. Rapid and automated technology for the isolation and purification of antibodies against proteins is being used widely to study their structural localization within cells. Also, technology for the rapid comparison of protein sequences within and across species is helping to provide valuable information about their potential function. However, because it may be difficult to predict the function of a protein based on homology to other proteins or even from their three-dimensional structure, it may be necessary to attempt to determine the various components of protein complexes or even cellular structures before their true function becomes apparent.

2.5.3   Transcriptomics

Functional genomics is also being enhanced by the emergence of powerful technologies which allow the analysis of the patterns of messenger RNA transcription of as many as 100,000 genes in a single experiment (Figure 2.5). Investigations of the "transcriptome" of cells in this way will make it possible to investigate the difference between gene expression in

Figure 2.5   MICROARRAY (DNA CHIP) TECHNOLOGY *(see color plate at end of book)* In this experiment human DNA has been incorporated into a series of microchips. To establish which genes are activated when a particular cell line is transformed by Epstein-Barr (EB) virus, total RNA was extracted from the transformed cells and converted to complementary DNA (cDNA); in this process the cDNA was labeled with a fluorescent dye (Cy3). The labelled cDNA was then applied to the chip. The colour signals vary according to the activity of the genes in the cell line. Each chip shows a doublet in one corner, called Cy3 landing lights, which are simply to orientate the position of the genes on the chip.

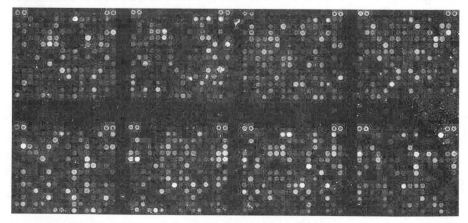

(Figure supplied by the courtesy of AT Merryweather-Clarke, C Langford, D Vetrie and KJH Robson, Weatherall Institute of Molecular Medicine, Oxford, United Kingdom)

various tissues and to analyse the variability of expression during different phases of disease. Microarray technology of this kind can also identify different classes of proteins, those bound to the membrane or those which are secreted, through the localization of their messenger RNAs (Lockhart and Winzler, 2000).

2.5.4   Gene regulation

So far there is only a primitive understanding of how genes are regulated. The key regulatory sequences for some genes have been identified and the actions of a wide range of different proteins that bind to DNA, and which are involved in the activation or repression of genes, have been characterized. However, there is very little information about the bigger picture of how batteries of genes are coordinated within cells and organisms. Because vital regulatory functions have been conserved across many species during evolution, much of this work will involve comparisons of the genomes of a variety of different species, ranging from fruitflies to humans. For example, invaluable information about such fundamental processes as the regulation of the cell cycle, essential to a better understanding of the genesis of cancer, has already been obtained for humans by comparisons with similar processes in yeast.

It is now possible selectively to inactivate or "knock-out" any particular gene in mice bred for this purpose, and this is proving an extremely valuable approach to defining gene function and regulation. For example, it has been possible to determine the functions of many of the effectors of the immune system and regulators of the early steps of haemopoiesis in this way. A variety of computer-based algorithms are also being developed to facilitate the identification of regulatory sequences.

As well as trying to understand the regulation and interaction of individual genes, a broader appreciation of the structural organization of the genome at different stages of development may have important consequences for understanding the mechanisms of human disease. For example, the genomes of many animals are compartmentalized, as reflected by packaging into either transcriptionally competent or silent regions, a process which starts early during embryonic development. It seems to reflect, at least in part, the degree of methylation of DNA. Recently developed techniques are allowing the methylation state of large regions of the genome to be analysed at different stages of development and in various disease states, particularly those involving development of the nervous system.

2.5.5   Bioinformatics

The huge databases that are emerging from this field, encompassing both sequence variation and expression of genes, and the structure of their protein products, will require major developments in computational biology for their analysis and interpretation in functional terms. And, as information of this type amasses, it will be necessary to develop sophisticated algorithms, forms of computer modelling and completely new fields of theoretical biology to attempt to interpret these data in terms of the complexities of how genes and their proteins interact one with another (Hasty et al., 2001).

2.6   THE GENOMES OF OTHER ORGANISMS

2.6.1   Introduction

To reap the full benefits of the human genome project and its aftermath for human biology and medicine, and for the most effective application of the new technology that will follow work in this field, it was equally vital that the genomes of other organisms were sequenced and studied in much the same way as the human genome. Indeed, for the improvement of the health of the developing countries the pathogen genome project may be of more immediate benefit. Work in this field is already well advanced.

2.6.2   The pathogen genome project

Coincident with the human genome project there has been extremely rapid progress both in the public and private sectors in different pathogen genome projects (Fraser et al., 2000). Already over 30 genomes have been sequenced or partially sequenced from important bacteria or parasites, and it is estimated that over the next two to four years more than 100 further species will be studied in this way (Box 2.3). Many viral genomes have also been sequenced.

The development of rapid sequencing strategies has made it possible to identify nearly all the protein-coding regions in prokaryotic genomes with confidence. Indeed, computational gene finders and various modelling techniques are now able routinely to find more than 99% of coding regions and RNA genes, and some progress is being made towards the identification of many of these genes. Using microarray technology it is possible to analyse the expression of batteries of microbial or parasite genes at different phases of infection and hence to define virulence determinants and to understand how pathogens "sense" their environments

Box 2.3   THE PATHOGEN GENOME PROJECT —
EXAMPLES OF SEQUENCING PROJECTS

Completed Genomes

Organism	Disease	Genome Size	Sequencing Institution	Funding*	Publication Year
Haemophilus influenzae	Meningitis, pneumonia	1.83 Mb	TIGR	TIGR	1995
Saccharomyces cerevisiae (budding yeast)	–	13 Mb	International consortium	EC, NHGRI, Wellcome Trust, McGill University, RIKEN	1996
Mycobacterium tuberculosis	Tuberculosis	4.4 Mb	Sanger Centre, Institut Pasteur	Wellcome Trust	1998
Campylobacter jejuni	Diarrhoeal disease	1.64 Mb	Sanger Centre	Beowulf Genomics	2000
Escherichia coli 0157 (two strains)	Food poisoning	5.5 Mb	Univ. of Wisconsin/ Japanese consortium	NHGRI, NIAID, Univ. of Wisconsin/ Japanese Society for Promotion of Science	2000
Vibrio cholerae	Cholera	4.0 Mb	TIGR	NIAID	2000
Mycobacterium leprae	Leprosy	3.26 Mb	Sanger Centre	The New York Community Trust/ Institute Pasteur	2000
Neisseria meningitidis	Bacterial meningitis	2.27 Mb	TIGR/ Sanger Centre	Chiron Corp/ Wellcome Trust	2000
Streptococcus pneumoniae	Pneumonia	2.20 Mb	TIGR	TIGR/ NIAID/MGRI	2001
Yersinia pestis	Plague	4.65 Mb	Sanger Centre	Beowulf Genomics	2001
Salmonella typhi (CT18)	Typhoid fever	4.5 Mb	Sanger Centre	Wellcome Trust	2001

Genomes in Progress

Organism	Disease	Genome Size	Sequencing Institutions	Funding
Plasmodium falciparum	Malaria	30 Mb	Malaria Genome Consortium	Wellcome Trust, NIAID, Burroughs Wellcome Fund, US Dept of Defence

Box 2.3	THE PATHOGEN GENOME PROJECT —
cont'd	EXAMPLES OF SEQUENCING PROJECTS

Genomes in Progress

Organism	Disease	Genome Size	Sequencing Institutions	Funding
Leishmania major (Friedlin)	Leishmaniasis	33.6 Mb	Sanger Centre, European consortium, SBRI	Beowulf Genomics European Commission, NIH
Trypanosoma brucei	African sleeping sickness	25 Mb	TIGR, Sanger Centre, TDR *T. brucei* genome network	NIAID, Wellcome Trust, Beowulf Genomics
Trypanosoma cruzi	Chagas Disease	–	TIGR. *T. cruzi* genome network	NIAID
Aspergillus fumigatus	Fungal infections	30–35 Mb	Sanger Centre, TIGR, Institut Pasteur Salamanca Univ., Nagasaki Univ.	NIH, NIAID, Wellcome Trust
Aspergillus nidulans	Model organism	30 Mb	Cereon Genomics	Cereon Genomics
Bacillus anthracis	Anthrax	4.5 Mb	TIGR	ONR/DOE NIAID/DERA

Sources: The Institute for Genome Research: (http://www.tigr.org)
The Sanger Centre (http://www.sanger.ac.uk)
* TIGR: The Institute for Genomics Research; EC: European Commission; NHGRI: National Human Genome Research Institute, USA; RIKEN: Institute of Physical and Chemical Research, Japan; NIAID: National Institute of Allergy & Infectious Diseases, USA; MGRI: Merck Genome Research Institute ; NIH: National Institutes of Health, USA; ONR: Office of Naval Research, USA ; DOE: Department of Energy, USA; DERA: Defence Evaluation & Research Agency, United Kingdom.

and evade host defence mechanisms. Studies of this type are already providing valuable information about how the genome of pathogens can change and adapt to the defence mechanisms of the host.

It has been estimated that, from the 100 or more projects for sequencing pathogen genomes, information should be obtained on over 300 000 genes. It is already clear that a significant number of them will be new and of unknown function. Hence they offer potential sources for developing completely new classes of vaccines or therapeutic agents.

In short, the process of annotation of pathogen genomes and of other organisms is proceeding very much along the lines outlined earlier for the human genome. Although it will take a long time to complete this venture it is clear that valuable information of great potential medical importance will emerge at each stage of the process.

2.6.3   The genomics of disease vectors

Progress is also being made towards an understanding of the genomics of vectors for important communicable diseases. For example, by early 2002, the entire genome sequence of the malaria-transmitting mosquito, *Anopheles gambiae*, will have been characterized by an international consortium (Hoffman et al., 2002). Extensive studies of the genomes of various strains of mosquitoes are providing information about mechanisms of gene transfer which may lead to the production of new forms with a reduced capacity for disease transmission (Enserink, 2001).

2.6.4   The genomes of the worm, fruitfly, yeast and various animals

One of the most important tools for identifying coding sequences as well as the regulatory regions of human and pathogen genes is the study of the genomes of other organisms. As mentioned below, the mouse genome is of particular importance in this respect. But valuable information can be obtained from the genomes of organisms in which the developmental patterns and genetics are particularly well defined, the nematode worm (*Caenorhabditis elegans*), the fruitfly (*Drosophila melanogaster*), and yeast (*Saccharomyces cerevisiae*), for example. The rat is a particularly important model for pharmaceutical research and for studying aspects of whole-animal physiology, brain function and complex disease. The simplicity of the zebrafish genome also has considerable potential for identifying and studying the function of genes which have been conserved during evolution. In both the public and private sectors, plans are also well advanced for sequencing other large vertebrate genomes, including the pig, cow, dog and chimpanzee.

2.6.5   The central importance of the mouse genome project

The importance of pursuing studies of the mouse genome for a better understanding of the functions and pathology of the human and pathogen genomes cannot be over emphasized (Justice, 2000; Nadeau, 2001). It has been known for some time that there are large chromosome segments which show conservation of correspondence of gene order (synteny) between mice and humans. A great deal is known already about mouse genetics and about the many diseases of mice which are similar to those of humans. And an increasingly wide variety of techniques are becoming available for modifying and studying the function of the mouse genome.

Mice offer particularly valuable experimental opportunities because it is possible to produce mutants using embryonic stem cell technology. In this way it is easy to "knock-out" individual genes, one gene at a time, and hence to examine their function. It is also possible to generate mutations using alkylating agents, and a variety of new recombinational systems are being investigated to establish larger genetic modifications. Several programmes are being developed to apply these techniques to study mouse chromosomes with particularly conserved synteny with human chromosomes as primary targets for physical and functional analysis.

Mice have many anatomical and physiological similarities to humans and suffer from many diseases which have human counterparts. Where these diseases do not exist they can be created by embryonic stem cell technology. Hence there are numerous examples of both monogenic and complex multigenic diseases in mice. These offer valuable opportunities for both the better understanding of the molecular pathology of disease and for testing novel therapeutic agents. They also provide models for investigating variation in the clinical phenotype of monogenic diseases. For example, it is possible to outbreed mice with single-gene disorders and to observe the change in the pattern of the disease. This is making it feasible to identify genes which can modify the course of these diseases and hence to find homologous modifiers of human disease.

2.6.6   Plant genomics

Although a detailed consideration of plant genomics and the genetic modification of crops was not within the remit of this Report, this rapidly growing field has important implications for improvements in human health.

A major international consortium was developed to map and sequence the genome of the model plant, *Arabidopsis thaliana,* and there are numerous projects, both in the private and public sector, directed at mapping and sequencing the genomes of a wide range of plant species. Although the primary aim of much of this work is to identify genes controlling important traits such as growth, fertility and disease resistance, there is increasing evidence that the genetic modification of plants may offer important possibilities for the delivery of vaccines or therapeutic agents for the control of human disease (Singer and Daar, 2001).

Apart from its value in the improvement of nutrition, the study of plant genomics and the modification of plant genomes also provides important information for the analysis of genomics and its applications in other organisms. For example, an understanding of how the interaction of a number of different genes can profoundly alter plant phenotypes, the growth and durability of tomatoes for example, has provided considerable insights into multigenic traits in animals and humans. The technology which is being applied for gene transfer in plants also has important lessons for the therapeutic uses of this approach in humans.

Some of the potential medical applications of pathogen and plant genomics are considered in Section 3.

2.7   SUMMARY

In short, the evolution of the genome projects and functional genomics will involve increasingly complex and expensive technology, data handling and theoretical biology, requiring multidisciplinary teams and interactions between academia and industry at a level that has hitherto not been possible. While the full benefits of these developments for medical practice may take many years to come to fruition, there will be undoubtedly a steady pipeline of new information and technologies which will have more immediate applications over the next few decades.

3. The Potential of Genomics for Health Care

3.1 Introduction

The study of disease at the cellular and molecular level has been evolving rapidly over the last 20 years and already a considerable amount of progress has been made. Hence, although the full implications for the further development of this field that may follow future progress in human and pathogen genomics are still uncertain, it is possible to make some cautious predictions about the clinical applications that may be generated along the way. They are based on the reasonable assumption that, if it has been possible to make considerable progress in human molecular genetics and pathology without knowledge of entire genome sequences and functional genomics, as this is obtained the field should move much faster.

3.2 Monogenic disease

Although there are some 5,000 diseases which are inherited in a simple Mendelian fashion, that is which result from mutations involving a single-gene, most of them are quite rare. Typical examples include inborn errors of metabolism, inherited haemoglobin disorders, cystic fibrosis and haemophilia. The global prevalence at birth of all single-gene disorders is about 10 per thousand. In Canada it has been estimated that, taken together, they may account for up to 40% of the work of hospital-based paediatric practice (Scriver, 1995).

By far the commonest monogenic diseases are those involving human haemoglobin, the thalassaemias and sickle cell disease and its variants, conditions which have a particularly high frequency in sub-Saharan Africa, the Mediterranean region, the Middle East, the Indian subcontinent and throughout southeast Asia (Figure 3.1). Approximately one in seven of the world's population are carriers for a gene for thalassaemia or a haemoglobin variant. There is increasing evidence that, as countries undergo the demographic transition (i.e. the change in a society from extreme poverty to a stronger economy, often associated by a transition in the pattern of diseases from malnutrition and infection to the intractable conditions of middle and old age, cardiovascular disease, diabetes, and cancer, for example), these conditions are posing an increasingly severe health burden. The evolution of thalassaemia in Cyprus is a good example. This condition was not identified in the island until 1944, when, after a major malaria eradication programme and accompanying improvements in public health, it became clear that among the children there was a common form of anaemia which was later identified as thalassaemia. By the early 1970s it was estimated that, if no steps were taken to control the disease, in about 40 years time the blood required to treat all the severely affected children would amount to 78,000 units per annum, 40% of the population would have to be blood donors, and the total cost of managing the disease would equal or exceed the Island's health budget (Weatherall and Clegg, 2001).

Between 1981 and 2000, 1112 genes in which mutations leading to monogenic disease were discovered as well as 94 genes involved in various forms of cancer (see Section 3.4) (Figure 3.2). A great deal is now known about the repertoire of the different kinds of mutations that underlie the molecular pathology of monogenic diseases and how they lead to a disease phenotype.

As knowledge of the monogenic diseases has accumulated it has become apparent that all of them show remarkable clinical heterogeneity, even within families with the same mutation. In the thalassaemia field, for example, it has been found that this effect is the result of heterogeneity of the underlying mutations, over 200 different mutations having been identified for one common form of thalassaemia, together with the action of

Figure 3.1 THE WORLD DISTRIBUTION OF THE β THALASSAEMIAS
The approximate number of births of affected babies each year are shown. For comparison, the approximate number of births of babies with sickle cell anemia (SS) each year in Africa is also shown.

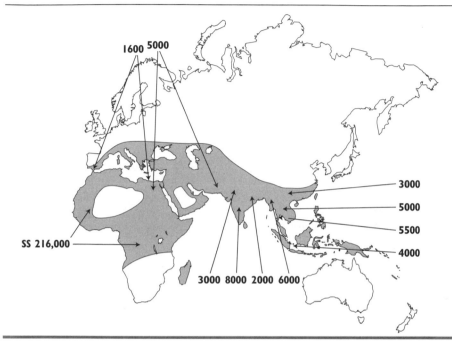

layer upon layer of modifier genes, which may reduce or increase the severity of the action of the mutant gene or which may act at a distance and modify some of the complications of the disease (Weatherall, 2001). Environmental factors may also modify the phenotype. These findings, which will undoubtedly be extended to most monogenic diseases, add a further dimension to the complexity of genetic counselling and predictive genetics.

This new genetic information, and the possible influence of environmental factors, has been already used widely for carrier detection, population screening and prenatal diagnosis, and has, in effect, revolutionized this aspect of medical practice in many developed countries. For example, through partnerships with groups in the USA and England, haematologists in Sardinia and Cyprus developed population screening programmes together with prenatal diagnosis for β thalassaemia, pioneering developments which have led to a dramatic reduction in the frequency of births of babies with this disorder. Much of the success of these programmes depended on the excellence of the public education initiative which pre-

Figure 3.2   THE PACE OF DISEASE GENE DISCOVERY AND THE MOLECULAR CHARAC-
TERIZATION OF CLINICAL DISORDERS (1981–2001).

A. The number of disease genes discovered so far is 1253. This number does not include most of the disease related genes identified as translocation gene-fusion partners in neoplastic disorders. Numbers in parentheses indicate disease related genes that are polymorphisms ("susceptibility genes")

B. The number of clinical diseases characterized (1746) does not include the many neoplastic disorders caused by translocation-related fusion genes.

(From Professor V.A. McKusick, Johns Hopkins University, Baltimore, MD, USA; refer also to Peltonen and McKusick, 2001)

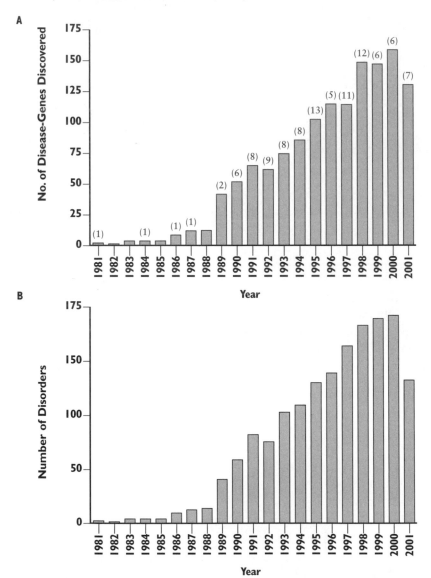

ceeded them. Comprehensive control programmes combining the best possible methods of prevention through carrier screening and counselling and treatment have been established in a number of countries in each WHO region. A group of WHO advisors supported by WHO collaborating centres have developed guidelines for the organization of such services in different countries (WHO, 2000). Extremely successful neonatal screening programmes for genetic disease have also been established, notably the pioneering development of this type in Montreal, Canada (Scriver, 1995). Neonatal screening is of particular value for diseases in which early prophylaxis or treatment is of value, sickle cell anaemia and phenylketonuria, for example.

Since by appropriate linkage studies and gene analyses it is now possible to isolate the genes for any monogenic disease, carrier detection and genetic counselling, backed up where appropriate by prenatal diagnosis, will become increasingly available for the control of these conditions. As more experience is gained of preimplantation diagnosis, that is DNA-based analysis of a few cells of fertilized ova obtained by in vitro fertilization, this is likely to become the method of choice for many couples at risk for having a child with a serious genetic disease. It has the particular advantage that it removes the need for termination of pregnancy.

Molecular genetic testing will be used for many purposes: accurate diagnosis; predictive testing for conditions without any current form of treatment such as Huntington's disease to allow individuals to make personal decisions for family planning; predictive testing leading to preventive treatment for such disorders as familial adenomatous polyposis; predispositional testing for conditions like familial breast cancer; carrier testing for recessive disorders like thalassaemia and Tay-Sachs disease; and, as outlined earlier, prenatal and neonatal testing.

Very few monogenic diseases can be cured at the moment although accurate diagnosis may lead to valuable symptomatic treatment, blood transfusion for thalassaemia and dietary restriction for phenylketonuria for example. The prospects for curing these conditions by gene therapy are considered in Section 3.9.

3.3   COMMUNICABLE DISEASE

There is growing evidence that a better knowledge of the genomics of pathogens and their vectors is likely to play a major role in the prevention and treatment of infectious disease.

Because of the relatively small size of their genomes, viruses were the first pathogens to be sequenced; the DNA sequence of the genome of a virus that infects bacteria was published by Sanger's team in 1977. Numerous viral genomes have now been sequenced and much is known about the way in which viruses infect cells, copy their genes and proteins by using the cell's machinery and raw materials, and package fresh copies into new viral particles that are able to infect other cells. From a knowledge of these processes at the molecular level it has been possible to design antiviral drugs which are able to disrupt the viral genome, interfere with protein synthesis, or block the spread of viruses from cell to cell.

Although the genomes of bacteria, parasites and disease vectors are very much more complex than those of viruses, as outlined in Section 2 the application of the tools of functional genomics and proteomics is likely to provide invaluable new diagnostic agents and information about both the mechanisms of virulence and how pathogens evade host defence mechanisms, which will lead to the production of new vaccines and therapeutic agents. It will also offer new ways to explore the population genetics and ecology of infectious disease, research which may provide novel approaches to the prevention of these diseases.

A variety of diagnostic agents are being developed which are turning out to have particular value for the identification of organisms which are difficult to grow in culture. This work has been facilitated by the use of the polymerase chain reaction (PCR), which allows the rapid amplification of small quantities of DNA or RNA. This approach is already finding a variety of invaluable uses in the diagnosis and control of infectious disease. For example, it allows the activity of infection due to hepatitis C virus to be monitored and assessed both before and during treatment and, as discussed in Section 5, it is proving of value in the diagnosis of several common parasitic and viral diseases.

Knowledge of the particular patterns of gene expression in pathogens, and the definition of virulence genes, is already starting to provide new targets for drug therapy. For example, such knowledge has led to the identification of a new class of antimalarial drugs which may be effective against multidrug resistant strains of *Plasmodium falciparum* (Box 3.1).

Similar approaches are also being directed at the development of new vaccines (Letvin et al., 2001). The pathogen genome has already yielded vaccine candidates against *Neisseria meningitidis*, group B, an important cause of meningitis. Using the entire genome sequence of a virulent strain, over 500 cell surface-expressed or secreted proteins were identified; the

Box 3.1   Fosmidomycin — Demonstrating the Potential of Genomic Knowledge for Application to Health Problems of Developing Countries

It is not often that a drug development process is as rapid or involves as many different players from across the globe as has been the case with the antimalarial candidate, fosmidomycin, which currently is undergoing proof of concept study. The story of fosmidomycin provides a clear demonstration of how the knowledge generated from genome sequencing projects could offer immediate and exciting opportunities for combating health care problems of the developing world.

Through computational analysis of the sequence data of the malarial parasite, *Plasmodium falciparum*, which is being generated by the Malaria Genome Project and released freely into public databases as it is produced, researchers working at the Justus Liebig University in Giessen, Germany made an important discovery. They found that the parasite utilized an enzymatic pathway called DOXP, which is present throughout the plant and bacteria kingdoms, but absent in humans. They realized that a drug, called fosmidomycin, had been developed by a Japanese company in the 1970s to target this very pathway which was crucial for the survival of the malarial parasite but absent from the biochemistry of humans. Fosmidomycin had never been marketed, despite good tolerance even at high doses, since it was not found to be effective against recurrent urinary infections - the purpose for which it had been originally developed. The group immediately tested fosmidomycin on mouse models of malaria, and found it to be a highly effective antimalarial agent.

Recognizing the potential of drugs targeting the DOXP pathway, the Justus Liebig group founded a start-up company (Jomaa Pharmaka) to develop therapeutic agents. In the meantime, initial clinical trials of fosmidomycin have already been completed in Thailand and Gabon, and the results have been encouraging. WHO, UNDP and World Bank Tropical Diseases Research (TDR) programme is helping to coordinate the oversight and monitoring of these trials and further studies to explore the activity of this drug are planned in Thailand in 2002. It is remarkable to note that, in the case of fosmidomycin, the path from the laboratory investigation to the initial clinical trials of this antimalarial candidate has been completed in less than 2 years, thanks to the power of bioinformatics and the availability of fundamental genomic knowledge in the public domain.

References

Jomaa H, Wiesner J, Sanderbrand S, Altincicek B, Weidemeyer C, Hintz M et al. (1999). Inhibitors of the nonmevalonate pathway of isoprenoid biosynthesis as antimalarial drugs. *Science* 285:1573–1576.

Stanford Genome Technology Centre. *The Malaria Genome Project* (Accessed at http://www-sequence.stanford.edu/group/malaria/ Jan 16, 2002)

corresponding DNA sequences were cloned and expressed in bacteria. Of the putative targets, over half were expressed successfully and used to immunize mice. From this large screening procedure two highly conserved vaccine candidates emerged.

A variety of related approaches towards the development of vaccines are being explored (Orme et al., 2001). Clinical trials of a vaccine against tuberculosis have already started using a combination of bacillus Calmette-Guérin (BCG) and a booster consisting of a vaccinia virus engineered to produce antigen 85, a protein which is synthesised by the tuberculosis bacterium, *Mycobacterium tuberculosis*. Another promising candidate for a vaccine against tuberculosis follows the observation that the intramuscular injection of a fragment of DNA encoding a so-called heat shock protein from a bacterium which is related to *M. tuberculosis* protects mice from the disease and, remarkably, seems to cure those that have been infected. Several promising DNA-based vaccines for the prevention of malaria are undergoing preliminary clinical testing. Recently the first trial of a pre-erythrocytic vaccine to show significant protection against natural *P. falciparum* infection has been reported (Bojang et al., 2001). The vaccine, RTS,S/ASO2, which consists of proteins derived from both the malarial parasite and hepatitis B virus, was formulated with a novel adjuvant (ASO2).

These examples are only a few of the ways in which genomics and related advances in the biological science are being used to develop vaccines. Different approaches are utilizing new information derived from knowledge of the immune system, including the network of cells known as dendritic cells which are able to sense different microbial stimuli and pass on this information to lymphocytes (white blood cells), and how the system's memory of antigens that it encounters is controlled. In the long-term it is hoped to develop ways of both boosting and prolonging responses to vaccine antigens.

Pathogen genomics will also be a valuable acquisition to the study of the population genetics, dynamics and ecology of infectious disease. Work in this field should provide valuable information about the movement of infectious diseases within populations, and anticipate the emergence of epidemics and of "new" or virulent forms of known infections; current examples include variant Creutzfeldt-Jakob disease, virulent forms of the bacterium *Escherichia coli* which causes food poisoning, new strains of influenza virus, hantaviruses, and human sleeping sickness, all of which seem to be increasing in different populations at the present time.

Progress is also being made towards a novel approach to a well-tried method for the prevention of communicable disease, that is, vector control. The discovery that transposons, stretches of DNA that can insert new genes into the genome, can be used to introduce genes into the genomes of mosquitoes, and reduce their ability to transmit malaria, is a promising example of this new approach (Enserink, 2001).

Genomics will also be applied to obtain a better understanding of variability in host response to infectious disease. Over recent years considerable progress has been made in identifying a variety of of gene families which are involved in modifying susceptibility to malaria. Similar progress has been made towards an understanding of variable susceptibility to other infections. For example, a mutation in a chemokine receptor, which is one of the receptors whereby HIV gains access to cells, is associated with marked resistance to AIDS. Work of this type has important practical applications. For example, once it was found that a structural alteration in a chemokine receptor results in relative resistance to infection with HIV, a search was initiated for chemokine analogues that could be used for inhibiting the entry of the virus into cells and hence for the treatment of AIDS. Genes, or families of genes, have also been discovered which provide at least some protection to other infections, including tuberculosis, hepatitis and several common parasitic illnesses in addition to malaria. In mice, genetic systems have been characterized which modify response to vaccines. These applications are discussed in more detail in Section 5.

This work on disease susceptibility will expand and plans are already advanced for developing genome-wide searches for identifying more genes that influence individual susceptibility to infectious agents. Furthermore, it is likely that there will be a better understanding of the mechanisms of variable host immune response to infection. In other words, understanding natural protective mechanisms against infectious agents should point to more logical ways of treating infectious disease.

Despite some remarkable successes in the control and treatment of communicable disease, these conditions are an everpresent threat to every country of the world; resistant or "new" organisms appear regularly. As knowledge of these conditions stems from pathogen genomics it will have to be incorporated into the classical approaches of public health and epidemiology which have been so successful in the past in controlling many infectious killers. And as the field evolves, at every stage the costs and efficacy of new diagnostic, preventive and therapeutic agents will have to be carefully assessed in comparison with more conventional approaches to the control of these diseases.

3.4   CANCER

Some of the most spectacular progress in the application of molecular and cell biology to the study of human disease has been made in the cancer field (Livingston and Shivdasani, 2001). These advances reflect the amalgamation of knowledge obtained from classical epidemiology, cytogenetics (the study of chromosomes), cell biology and tumour virology. It is now clear that most cancers result from the acquisition of mutations in a family of "housekeeping genes" called "cellular oncogenes." These mutations may result from a lifelong exposure to external carcinogens or from the powerful oxidants which are being produced continually as part of normal body metabolism. Alternatively, oncogenes may be activated or deregulated due to specific chromosomal abnormalities, many of which had been observed by researchers in the cancer field for many years. Oncogenes are involved in many of the basic functions of a cell. For example, they are responsible for responses to external regulatory signals, for the ability to recognise when DNA is defective and hence to act as a check so that the cell does not go into a division cycle and pass on the defect to its progeny, and the many and complex processes of DNA repair. Many cancers require the acquisition of multiple oncogene mutations before the disease is fully expressed.

While most of the common forms of cancer appear to result from mutations of oncogenes which are acquired as we get older, there is a much rarer group which is associated with a strong family history of cancer. Many of these conditions appear to result from mutations of a family of genes called "tumour suppressor genes." There is strong evidence that in many cases, when a mutated allele of a tumour suppressor gene is inherited, a further mutation of the normal allele is required before a tumour is generated. Some examples of these rare familial cancers and the genes involved are shown in Box 3.2.

These remarkable findings are leading to some fundamental rethinking about the prevention and management of cancer. They suggest, for example, that it should be possible to classify particular tumours according to the expression of different sets of genes. Using microarray technology it has already been found that this is the case for certain cancers of the blood or breast and that different patterns of gene expression carry different prognoses. It is hoped, therefore, that cancer therapy will change from the blunderbuss approach of destroying both malignant and healthy cells by radiotherapy or chemotherapy to treatment that is more functionally directed. For example, as mentioned above, in the case of some cancers, major chromosomal changes, including translocations resulting in the exchange of pieces of chromosome with one another, give rise to disordered oncogene function. Recently it has been possible to manufacture

Box 3.2   TUMOUR SUPPRESSOR GENES ASSOCIATED WITH FAMILIAL CANCER
SYNDROMES

Gene	Associated Inherited Cancer
RB1	Retinoblastoma
APC	Familial adenomatous polyposis coli Gardener syndrome
NF-1	Neurofibromatosis 1
NF-2	Neurofibromatosis 2
BRCA 1	Familial breast and ovarian cancer
BRCA 2	Inherited breast and pancreatic cancer
WT-1	WAGR Syndrome (Wilm's tumour, aniridia and abnormalities of urogenital development)
MEN-1	Multiple endocrine neoplasia
EXT-1	Hereditary multiple exostoses
TSC-1	Tuberous sclerosis
TP53	L1-Fraumeni Syndrome. Widespread tumours of bone and organs
MSH2, *MLH1,* *Others*	Hereditary non-polyposis Colorectal cancer

Over 20 tumour suppressor genes have been identified. The mechanisms of action of many of them are known. According to Knudson's "two-hit" hypothesis, two inactivating mutations are required. In the case of retinoblastoma, for example, the first may either be inherited in the germ cell, or acquired as a somatic-cell mutation. The second mutation is always somatic. The mechanisms have been confirmed by demonstrating allele loss in tumour tissues.

a drug directed at a specific product of this kind of event, a tyrosine kinase that is produced at the site of a chromosome translocation in a common form of leukaemia (Druker and Lydon, 2000; Schindler et al., 2000). This agent has shown dramatic effects in destroying the leukaemia cell population and has also been found to be effective in other forms of cancer associated with abnormal tyrosine kinase activity. However, the recent report of emergence of cell populations which are resistant to this new agent due to the production of a variant kinase, is, though not surprising, a harsh reminder of how far we have to go, even in chemotherapy directed at the underlying molecular mechanisms of malignant transformation.

A great deal of work is being directed at discovering other ways to interfere with the activity of oncogene function in cancer and it seems very likely that, in the long-term, molecular approaches both to the classification of tumours and to their management will lead to considerable improvements in the control of cancer and its treatment.

Particularly in view of the continuing rise in deaths from tobacco-related cancers, well-tried public health measures will remain the most important approach to the prevention of these diseases for the foreseeable future. However, genomics is likely to play an increasingly important role in cancer prevention, and its new technologies will undoubtedly become integrated into epidemiological and public health practice.

In the case of the rare familial cancers(see Box 3.2), in which it has become possible to predict with a considerable degree of certainty the likelihood of an individual developing a particular cancer, DNA-based diagnostic approaches are becoming of great value. In effect, they enable individuals in affected families who are found not to carry the mutation to be relieved of further anxiety, while, at the same time, they make it possible for those who are carrying tumour suppressor gene mutations of this type to undergo careful surveillance or, when appropriate, prophylactic treatment. For example, those affected with the gene for familial adenomatous polyposis may consider undergoing surgery before they develop cancers of the colon.

It seems likely that genes which predispose towards common cancers will be identified through genome searches or related approaches and that this information may then be fed into public health programmes for the prevention of cancer. Many studies are examining the feasibility of the early identification of cancer by looking for oncogene mutations in cells shed into the bowel or sputum. However, all these fields are at an early stage of development and it is vital that adequate pilot studies are carried out before any of them are integrated into widespread population screening programmes for cancer. For example, there is now considerable evidence that the human papilloma virus (HPV) of a particular subtype is related to the development of cancer of the cervix. This has led to the possibility of screening based on the use of an HPV DNA probe in cervical cells. Currently, there is considerable uncertainty about whether this test could be widely adapted and its genuine value for the diagnosis of cervical cancer. Hence efforts are also being made to enhance the value of standard cytological analysis by the use of markers for particular oncogene mutations. This is a good example of the need for caution, detailed scientific analysis, and very careful preparatory pilot studies before embarking on any wide-scale cancer screening.

3.5   COMPLEX MULTIFACTORIAL DISEASE

It has been appreciated for a long time that many common killers or causes of chronic ill-health, heart disease, stroke, diabetes, the major psychoses, and so on, are the result of environmental factors and the effects of ageing, modified to some degree by our genetic make-up. Twin studies have suggested a variable genetic component, strong in late-onset diabetes but weaker in heart disease, for example. Similar observations have been made for the major psychoses, particularly schizophrenia and the bipolar affective disorders. There is also evidence that the same mechanisms may be involved in the generation of the common dementias, notably Alzheimer disease.

The aim of molecular genetics is to attempt to identify the different genes involved in variable susceptibility to environmental agents or the effects of ageing. The rationale of this approach, upon which much hope is pinned for the improvement of health care in the future, is that if variation in function of several different genes can combine to make an individual more prone to develop coronary artery disease or schizophrenia, for example, then it is likely that the products of these genes are related to the underlying pathology. If this is the case, identifying these genes and their products offers a direct approach to understanding the basic cause of these conditions, including how they are triggered by a variety of environmental factors. This information, in turn, should become of value to the pharmaceutical industry in developing agents which can be targeted at the basic cause of these conditions. In addition, once the genetic profile of individuals who are particularly susceptible to various environmental factors can be ascertained, it may be possible to focus public health measures for the prevention of these conditions much more effectively.

So far there has been some progress in determining a few of the genes involved in these multigenic systems, notably in the case of diabetes, coronary artery disease, Alzheimer disease, asthma, and others. Hitherto, most of these successes have stemmed from studies of candidate genes, that is selecting genes whose products are likely to play some role in vascular disease or diabetes, for example. The other method, extended family or population studies together with "total genome" searches using linkage markers, has so far been less successful. It has provided some evidence about susceptibility genes for insulin-dependent diabetes, both in mouse and man, and has disclosed some potential candidate genes for susceptibility to asthma. But there have been many failures.

Another approach to studying the genetics of common disease has been to look for the unusual forms of these diseases which are inherited in a simple Mendelian fashion. For example, monogenic forms of diabetes may account for up to 5% of all cases of the disease. At least five different genes have been found to cause these forms of diabetes. Similarly, studies of families in which individuals have an early onset of Alzheimer disease have led to the discovery of several of the genes involved. It is hoped that a better understanding of the genetic abnormalities in unusual families of this type may offer leads to the discovery of genes involved in the more common forms of these conditions.

However, the major hope for defining susceptibility genes for common disease lies in the new technology which is being developed as part of the Human Genome Project and functional genomics. As discussed in Section 2, a major effort is being made to map the human genome with markers for linkage studies, including SNPs and, more importantly, regions of DNA marked by haplotypes of these polymorphisms. Recently it has been found that humans have fewer SNP haplotypes than was suspected; 80% of a globally diverse set of chromosomes could be characterized by only three common ones. It has been suggested that disease-association studies may require the comparison of total genomes (Kwok, 2001).

Although many technical and computational difficulties remain and the extent to which these markers will facilitate gene finding is currently unclear, some recent developments are extremely encouraging. For example, using SNPs it has been possible to define a locus on chromosome 16 which confers susceptibility for developing Crohn's disease, a common inflammatory disease of the bowel (Lesage et al., 2000; Hugot at al., 2001). This gene, *NOD2-CARD15*, is part of a gene superfamily which act as intracellular receptors for pathogenic microbial components. Interestingly, it had long been suspected that this disease might have an infectious basis.

Using similar technology a genome-wide screen has been carried out for susceptibility genes for type 2 diabetes among Mexican Americans and a susceptibility locus which seems to be shared with North Europeans has been assigned to chromosome 2. Positional cloning has led to the identification of a gene which is a ubiquitously expressed member of the calpain-like cysteine protease family (Baier et al., 2000; Horikawa et al., 2000). The identification of this susceptibility gene for diabetes suggests that there may be a hitherto unidentified biochemical pathway involved in the regulation of glucose metabolism. Many other large-scale studies of this type are well advanced but because some of them are in the private sector it is not clear to what extent they have been successful. For example, because it is argued that gene finding of this kind may be facilitated in populations with limited numbers of founders, large-scale association strategies have been designed for the populations of Iceland, Sardinia, Finland and Estonia, all, in part at least, funded by the private sector (see Section 6).

Enough is therefore known about this new field of the role genetic factors in complex multifactorial diseases to suggest that a number of susceptibility genes will be identified and that this will lead to a better understanding of the underlying pathology of these common diseases and may well result in the identification of molecular targets for drug design. A word of caution is necessary however. Most of these conditions result from the action of environmental factors in the background of genetic susceptibility which probably reflects the action of a number of different genes. Identification of any one of these genes does not necessarily mean that it is a major player in the pathology of these conditions. Furthermore, many of these disorders are extremely heterogeneous and their pathology is complicated by the ill-understood changes of ageing.

While these issues have important implications for drug design, they are even more pertinent to the integration of genomic information for preventive medicine and public health. But it may be a very long time before widespread population screening for susceptibility for common disease becomes of genuine value. In the meantime it is vital that the more conventional approaches of epidemiology and public health, particularly as they relate to tobacco-induced diseases and other aspects of lifestyle, continue to be pursued with vigour. This is particularly important as there are still major uncertainties about the predictive role and cost of genomics for controlling common diseases.

The pursuit of an integrative approach of this kind is particularly germane in the field of mental disorders, which is predicted to become an increasingly important problem in the future. For example, in the case of the common bipolar affective disorders, an understanding of the role of rapid changes in environment and lifestyles compared with genetic susceptibility will require a close collaboration between psychiatry, the social sciences, epidemiology and genomics.

3.6   DEVELOPMENTAL ABNORMALITIES AND MENTAL RETARDATION

These disorders constitute an important part of paediatric practice throughout the world. The prevalence at birth is about 2–3%, though the prevalence of individual abnormalities vary between different countries. For example, neural tube defects are common in China, Egypt and Mexico, while cleft lip and palate is more frequent in Amerindian and Asian populations. The development of molecular genetics is already having a major impact on our understanding of the pathogenesis of some of these conditions.

The availability of new techniques in cytogenetics is leading to a much more precise analysis of chromosomal disorders as the basis for developmental defects. Techniques such as in situ hybridization with labelled DNA or RNA probes, especially fluorescent in situ hybridization (FISH) (Figure 3.3), are leading to the discovery of small, submicroscopic chromosomal abnormalities in patients with these types of disorders. For example, it has been found that submicroscopic deletions of the telomeres (chromosome ends) are associated with about 10% of previously unexplained cases of mild to severe mental retardation. And some of the monogenic disorders associated with skeletal malformation have been found to result from mutations in genes that are involved in regulation of various stages of development. Similarly, monogenic conditions which interfere with brain metabolism and development have been defined at the DNA level. The discovery of the *Hox* gene system, which is highly conserved throughout all vertebrate species, is also providing valuable new insights into the mechanisms of human development and its pathology.

This very active field of the genetic basis of developmental abnormalities and mental retardation is already producing important diagnostic and counselling information and is likely to contribute significantly to our knowledge of these conditions in the future. But, while progress is being made towards a better understanding of conditions that are monogenic or result from chromosome abnormalities, many of these conditions have a major environmental component and do not follow any obvious pattern of inheritance. As is the case for other complex diseases, these disorders may well require a genetic epidemiological approach for their clarification. Hopes for their prevention and management are based on identifying environmental causes, discovering genetic abnormalities of brain metabolism that are amenable to correction, and specific gene therapy, as discussed later in this section.

Figure 3.3 MULTICOLOUR FLUORESCENT *in situ* HYBRIDISATION (FISH) ANALYSIS OF CHROMASOMES *(see color plate at end of book)*

The upper figure shows a normal human male set of chromosomes. Each chromosome is identified by a different combination of fluorescent dyes attached to specific DNA fragments which bind to particular human chromosomes. This method allows the detection of inter-chromosomal rearrangements and other chromosomal abnormalities. Each chromosome can be identified by its particular colour. The lower figure shows the chromosomes of a gibbon, which has 38 chromosomes. These have been analysed using a human FISH probe. The multicoloured chromosomes show the remarkable interchromosomal rearrangements which have occurred during the divergence of humans and gibbons over 14 million years.

(Figure kindly supplied by Dr. Willem Rens and Professor Malcolm Ferguson-Smith).

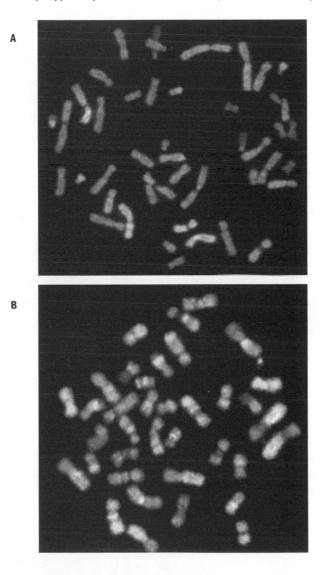

3.7   AGEING

The unpredicted increase in the relative proportion of the aged in many countries is producing major problems for their health services. These difficulties will be experienced by every country which has passed through the demographic transition and hence in which there is a major reduction of death in early life. Hitherto, the biology of ageing has been neglected. However, it is becoming clear that many of the common diseases of middle and old age are related to the ill-understood mechanisms that lead to the slow, insidious declines in structure and function observed in most organisms. Thus as well as work directed at the social and medical aspects of ageing, there is an urgent need for a better understanding of some of the biological mechanisms involved.

Unexpectedly, recent studies indicate that both the intrauterine and immediate postnatal environments may play a major role in later development and even susceptibility to diseases of middle and later life, notably cardiovascular disease and diabetes (Barker, 2001). These observations may have profound consequences for the health of large populations of the world. There is now the opportunity to combine classical epidemiological approaches with genome searches to attempt to distinguish between the roles of the fetal environment and genetic constitution in causing the high frequency of heart disease and diabetes in many of the world's populations.

The postgenome era is also seeing the development of technology which will provide important new insights into the biology and mechanisms of ageing (Novartis Foundation Symposium, 2001). From work based on knowledge of the genomes of fruit flies and worms it has become apparent that at least part of the ageing process may be related to the declining ability of physiological defence mechanisms against the damaging effects of both endogenous and exogenous oxidants on DNA and proteins. Furthermore, there is at least preliminary evidence that certain genes which are involved in modifying the ageing process may have been conserved throughout evolution. For example, it has been found that allelic variants of a gene of this kind called *daf2* in the nematode have counterparts in the fruit fly, and there is also evidence that comparable genes may be operative in mice. Clearly, therefore, we now have the tools with which to search for other critical "geromodulators" of this kind and to study how variation in their function may be related to some of the structural changes and even the pathology associated with ageing.

Since it seems likely that many of the diseases of middle and old age, such as heart disease, cancer and others, may at least, in part, reflect similar ageing mechanisms, work on the genetic and biological basis of ageing should provide valuable information about the pathogenesis of many common diseases.

3.8   Pharmacogenomics

It has been known for a long time that there is wide individual variation in response to drugs, and that drug toxicity or efficacy has a genetic component (Box 3.3). For example, the red blood cells of millions of people throughout the world are deficient in the enzyme glucose-6-phosphate dehydrogenase (G6PD). This causes serious haemolytic anaemia in response to antimalarial or other oxidant drugs, or certain foods. The acetylation polymorphism which results in the rapid or slow inactivation of the antituberculous drug, isoniazid, is another good example of this phenomenon.

It is widely believed that one of the benefits of the genome programmes will be the identification of numerous polymorphisms in metabolic pathways involving drug metabolism and action, and that this information will provide a completely new approach to therapeutics, with the dose of a drug being individually tailored to the particular biochemical networks of the patient (Roses, 2000). There have even been suggestions that within the next 20 years doctors will have computerized printouts of their patients' genetic make-up such that they will be able to prescribe drugs in an individualized way. It is far too early to determine the extent to which these hopes will turn out to be valid and whether this approach will be cost-effective.

In populations in which there is a high frequency of side-effects due to genetic susceptibility to a drug that is used to treat a common disease, genetic screening is undoubtedly worthwhile. For example, this is already practised in some countries in which G6PD deficiency is particularly common and where it is frequently necessary to prescribe certain antimalarial drugs. Genetic screening of this type will also be important in any population in which genetic variants that result in reduced efficiency of drugs used to treat common diseases are found frequently. For example, recent studies in West Africa suggest that this approach may be valuable in the case of lack of response to anti-HIV drugs (see Section 5).

The same principles apply to infectious agents also. The metabolic pathways whereby bacteria, parasites or other pathogens become resistant

Box 3.3   PHARMACOGENOMICS

Gene	Drug	Clinical consequence
Drug metabolism		
NAT-2	Isoniazid, hydralazine, procainamide, sulphonamides	Neuropathy, lupus erythematosus
CYP2D6	β blockers, antidepressants, codeine, debrisoquine, antipsychotics, many others	Arrhythmias, dyskinesia with antipsychotics, narcotic effects, changes in efficacy, many others
CYP2C9	Tolbutamide, phenytoin, non-steroidal anti-inflammatories	Anticoagulant effects of warfarin modified
RYR-1	Halothane and other anaesthetics	Malignant hyperthermia
Protection against oxidants		
G6PD	Primaquine, sulphonamides, acetanilide, others	Haemolytic anaemia
Drug Targets		
ACE	Captopril, enalapril	Modifies response to treatment of cardiac failure, hypertension, renal disease
HERG	Quinidine	Cardiac arrhythmia (long QT syndrome)
HKCNE2	Clarithromycin	Drug-induced arrhythmia

Examples of genetic polymorphisms which cause unwanted effects of drugs or modification of response. Currently, arrays are being developed for the rapid identification of families of polymorphisms related to infection-defence genotypes, drug-metabolism genotypes, and many others. Although many polymorphisms associated with variations to drug response or toxicity have been defined, the bulk of variation of response to drugs follows a multifactorial pattern of inheritance.

The examples shown are as follows:

NAT-2: N-acetyltransferase

CYP: Cytochrome P450

RYR-1: Ryanidine receptor

G6PD: Glucose-6-phosphate dehydrogenase

ACE: Angiotensin converting enzyme

HERG and HKCNE2 are potassium channels

Reference: Modified from Evans and Relling (1999).

to therapy has been a subject of intense study over recent years and at least some of the mechanisms are already known. Once the genes involved are determined it may prove cost-effective to screen pathogen populations using DNA-based technology as part of epidemiological studies to assess the most effective forms of therapy for common communicable diseases in populations.

3.9   GENE THERAPY

The term "gene therapy" is used to cover a variety of approaches for the treatment of disease by altering the genetic make-up of cells, organs, or individuals (Somia and Verma, 2000). There are two main approaches for achieving this end.

First, germ-line gene therapy involves the introduction of foreign DNA into a fertilized egg, or otherwise altering the genetic constitution of an egg. In this case, the "foreign" gene is distributed among all the tissues of the developing fetus, including the germ cells, and therefore the genetic alteration would be passed on to future generations. Although an attempt of this kind, involving mitochondrial DNA, has been reported from the private sector in the USA, in most countries this approach is currently banned.

The second technique, somatic-cell gene therapy, involves the modification of the genome of cells of individual organs or tissues. In this case, the inserted or altered genes only survive for the lifespan of the individual and are not passed on to their offspring. Most ethics committees have agreed that the procedure is no different in principle to organ transplantation. Although somatic-cell gene therapy is the subject of intense research, there have, to date, been very few successes.

In an attempt to control or cure monogenic or other diseases, somatic-cell gene therapy involves the isolation of the appropriate gene and its regulatory regions, developing an approach for inserting it into a reasonably large recipient cell population (to ensure sufficient cells receive the gene), and ensuring that the procedure has no deleterious effects on the patient. The major challenges revolve around the transfer of DNA (transfection) to a sufficient number of cells to obtain a therapeutic response and, once this has been achieved, in maintaining the function of the inserted gene for a reasonable period of time. A variety of methods have been used, including introducing the appropriate DNA by physical means, packaging it in fatty particles called liposomes, or, most effectively, inserting it into viral vectors. Many viruses have been explored; among the most promising are members of the adenovirus and adeno-associated virus families. By a variety of ingenious approaches it has been possible to insert relatively large pieces of DNA into these viruses and, with the aid of helper-cell lines, to provide high enough titres to obtain a relatively efficient level of transfection. Currently, the most promising results are being obtained for genetic diseases in which the inserted gene does not need tight regulation or a high level of expression.

Many other approaches are being tried, including site-directed recombination, that is exchanging sections of genes, injecting naked DNA, and the development of artificial chromosomes (Ferber, 2001). For a few diseases, attempts are being made to reactivate genes that are only expressed in fetal life to take the place of their defective adult counterparts. This concept is of particular relevance to the genetic disorders of haemoglobin.

There is steady progress on all these fronts and it seems likely that somatic-cell gene therapy will play an increasing role in the management of monogenic disease although there may still be many years of frustration before this becomes routine clinical practice. Another major problem which will have to be faced before this happens is that some important monogenic diseases are expressed early during development, particularly those involving the brain and other parts of the nervous system. For this reason, thoughts are already turning to the possibility of intrauterine gene therapy. But although this may become a possibility, it seems far too soon to be pursuing this line of research, certainly before the results of gene therapy using adult cells or tissues are more successful.

It is likely that gene therapy will make an impact on clinical practice for more short-term objectives before the treatment of monogenic disease is fully established. Already, clinical trials are underway with the objective of modifying the genetic constitution of arterial walls to interfere with the thrombosis of arterial grafts. A variety of methods are being explored to modify the abnormal function of oncogenes or to otherwise target drugs to treat cancer, and similar approaches are being applied to the control of many other common diseases (Box 3.4).

3.10   STEM CELL THERAPY

Stem cells are cell populations which have retained the ability to differentiate down different pathways in response to appropriate regulatory agents. Currently, stem cells can be obtained from some adult and fetal tissues, umbilical cord blood, early embryos, and theoretically at least, from other adult cells. It appears that the stem cells from many of these sources

Box 3.4   Clinical Trials in Gene Therapy Carried Out in 2001

Vector	Number of trials	Examples of diseases being treated
Viral		
Retrovirus	157	Many cancers, AIDS, severe combined immunodeficiency, rheumatoid arthritis, graft-versus-host disease, multiple sclerosis, osteodysplasia, haemophilia
Adenovirus	132	Many cancers, peripheral artery disease, cystic fibrosis, Canavan disease
Pox virus	35	Many cancers
Adeno-associated virus	7	Prostate cancer, cystic fibrosis, haemophilia B
Non-viral		
Lipofection	57	Many cancers, cystic fibrosis, coronary artery disease, restenosis
Naked DNA	47	Many cancers, peripheral artery disease, coronary artery disease, peripheral neuropathy, open bone fractures
RNA transfer	5	Many cancers
Gene gun	4	Melanoma, sarcoma

A recent compilation of gene therapy trials currently being carried out, mainly for non-genetic (non-monogenic) disorders. Based on Ferber (2001).

have limited plasticity regarding the cell lines into which they will develop and it is only those derived from human embryos that seem to have a toti-potential capacity.

Several groups have isolated embryonic stem cells from the inner cell mass of "spare" embryos from fertility clinics. These cells were then allowed to develop to the blastocyst stage. Cell lines have been cultured from the blastocyst for 4–5 months without differentiation, during which time they maintained the potential to form all of the main groups of embryonic germ layers. These early observations have raised the hope that it will be possible to derive a variety of cell types from stem cells, including those of the nervous system, heart, pancreas, cartilage, blood, liver, skin, bone, retina and skeletal muscle.

The availability of cells of this type could have considerable potential for the treatment of disease (Kaji and Leiden, 2001). Currently, this research is at a very early stage but the hope is that by studying embryonic stem cells more will be learnt about the properties of stem cells such that it may even be possible to treat the nuclei of adult cells so that they could be induced to differentiate into specific tissue types. Unfortunately, these approaches have been called "therapeutic cloning." It should be emphasized that this work is not directed at cloning in the sense of developing individuals of identical genetic make-up, but, rather, at learning how to isolate and grow cells with the potential to differentiate into specific tissues for therapeutic purposes.

One of the major difficulties which will have to be overcome before stem cell therapy becomes a genuine possibility is immune rejection of the products of cell lines derived from different individuals. This problem will have to be approached, either by some form of genetic engineering of particular cell populations or by learning how to transfer nuclei from an individual who is to be treated into an egg from which the nucleus has been removed, a procedure more akin to genuine reproductive cloning. The legal and ethical issues relating to research in this field are considered in Sections 6 and 8.

3.11   PLANT GENOMICS AND HUMAN HEALTH

Because this Report focuses on the medical applications of human and pathogen genomics it is beyond its scope to consider in detail the field of plant genomics. However, it is important to outline the role of this extremely important field, particularly as it relates to the objectives of WHO.

Over the next 25 years, the world's population is likely to increase by about 2.5 billion people, with the bulk of this projected growth occuring in developing countries. Food requirements in the developing world are expected to double by 2025. However, there has been a decline in the annual rate of increase in cereal production, so that the present yield is below the rate of population increase. It has been estimated that about 40% of plant productivity in parts of Africa and Asia, and about 20% in the developed world, is lost to pathogens; approximately one third of the losses are due to viral, fungal and bacterial pathogens, while the remainder is due to insects and nematodes. Much of this loss occurs after plants are fully grown, leading to the wasteful use of both land and the world's limited water supplies.

The genetic modification of plants has enormous potential for improving the world's food supplies and the health of its communities. Plant genomics is well advanced and many of the methods that are being used to construct genetically modified (GM) plants follow similar principles to those outlined earlier for gene transfer in humans and animals. For example, vectors have been designed to deliver transgenic DNA into the plant chloroplast genome by recombination; the lack of chloroplasts in pollen contributes to the environmental containment of the transgenes. Alternatively, trait and plant selection genes can be introduced on separate DNA fragments.

The main aims of GM plant technologies are to enhance the nutritional value of crop species and to confer resistance to pathogens. There have already been major successes in both these ventures. For example, by ingenious genetic engineering it has been possible to produce a strain of rice which is able to produce provitamin A, a development with great potential for reducing the rates of eye disease and infection world-wide. It should also be possible to engineer pathways for the production of other vitamins in plants (Ye et al., 2000). A number of disease-resistant crops have also been produced by genetic manipulation. Although concerns remain about the safety of GM crops, and a great deal more research is required, there is no doubt that this field has enormous potential for improving the nutritional status and health of the world's populations.

Plant genetics also has more direct potential for the control of disease in humans. In particular, by genetically modifying plants it is hoped that it will be possible to produce edible vaccines which are cheaper than conventional vaccines and which can be grown or freeze dried and shipped anywhere in the world. A promising example is the production of hepatitis B surface antigen in transgenic plants for oral immunization. Similarly, a trial of a recombinant hepatitis B vaccine that has been incorporated into potatoes is underway. Work is also well advanced for the production of vaccines against cholera, measles and human papilloma virus which, as discussed earlier, is implicated in the generation of cancer of the cervix.

If these new ventures are successful, research in this field could play a major role in disease control, particularly in the developing countries.

3.12   FORENSIC MEDICINE

Genomics is already making a major impact on forensic medicine. Because our DNA contains many regions which are highly variable in their structure, no two people are alike except for identical twins with respect to the patterns produced when it is treated with enzymes that cut the DNA into small pieces. This enables forensic scientists to produce so-called DNA fingerprints (Figure 3.4). As well as from blood, DNA can be obtained from body fluids and many tissues including bone and it is relatively stable, often over many years. For these reasons, DNA fingerprinting has become a major tool in forensic medicine. It has the added advantages that very

Figure 3.4   DNA FINGERPRINTING

DNA is cut by enzymes and the fractions separated and analysed by probes for particularly highly variable regions of the genome. The fractions are separated by their size. The figure shows the DNA from four different individuals, K, G, A and E. The DNA of K, G and A is run in duplicate to show the remarkable reproducibility of these patterns. The size of the bands is measured in kilobases (kb) and is assessed by running appropriately sized markers as indicated.

(Figure kindly supplied by Professor Sir Alec Jeffreys.)

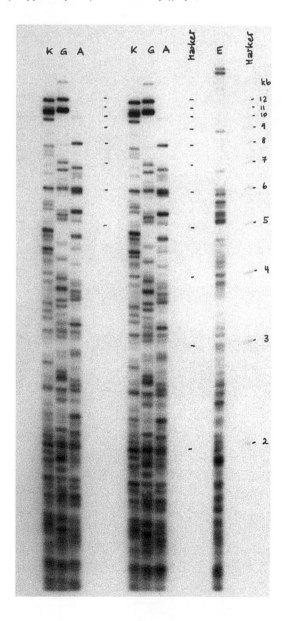

small quantities are required for identification purposes and samples can be obtained non-invasively from suspects, by the use of a simple mouthwash or swab for example.

3.13   BIOTECHNOLOGY

So far, the product pipeline from molecular genetics for the biotechnology industry has been limited. A few genes for monogenic diseases have been patented and diagnostic kits developed, but on the whole monogenic disease has been of little interest to industry. The gene probes required for the extensive diagnostic studies and prenatal diagnosis that have been used in many countries to control the haemoglobin disorders have been developed in academia and made freely available throughout the scientific community. Some diagnostic agents of value for the identification of pathogens have been developed commercially, but so far there have only been a limited number of important therapeutic agents produced in this way. Important examples include recombinant hepatitis B vaccine, erythropoietin, insulin, growth hormone, and tissue plasminogen activator (TPA).

These are early days however. It has been estimated that successful drug therapy currently is directed at fewer than 500 targets. Considering that the human genome contains some 30,000 genes, it is possible that its study could lead to at least 3,000 to 5,000 potential new targets for therapy. Currently, predominant candidates include G protein-coupled receptor families and other receptors and related molecules, a wide range of enzymes including proteases, kinases and phosphatases, hormones, growth factors, chemokines, soluble receptors and related molecules, and many others. Exactly the same principles are being applied to the search for agents to interfere with key biochemical pathways in pathogens, based on information which is being obtained from the pathogen genome project.

3.14   BROADER ISSUES OF BIOLOGY

Genomics is already playing a major role in evolutionary biology. It is helping to explain the origins of biological diversity in the context of natural selection, information which may yield important information about why present-day human genotypes are ill-suited to new environments, and how this may contribute to many common diseases.

Studies of genome diversity indicate that each of us is unique. The genetic differences that exist between two individuals of different racial backgrounds are no greater than those between two individuals of the same race. Again these observations may have clinical application. For example, it has been found recently that different alleles of drug-metabolizing enzymes are more closely related to clusters defined by highly polymorphic DNA markers on the X chromosome than to different racial groups as assessed by the usual morphological criteria (Wilson et al., 2001). The small genetic differences between races as usually defined probably reflect biological adaptations to different environments over long periods of time. The more that is learnt about the individual uniqueness and diversity of human beings, the less the concepts of "race" seem to have any meaning.

3.15   Summary

Enough was known before the recent successes of the human, pathogen and vector genome projects to suggest that the study of disease at the level of molecules and cells was likely to have major benefits for medical practice. The rapid advances in genomics over the next few years will undoubtedly build on what has been achieved and have the potential to help to control some of the most intractable diseases of humankind.

4. Relevance and Time-Scale of Advances in Genomics for Global Health

Contents

4.1 Genomics in the context of current world health problems

The potential of the applications of genomics for improving global health has to be viewed in the context of the current problems of the provision of health care. These range from the spiralling costs of its delivery in developed countries, reflecting the intractable nature of many of the diseases of middle life and old age together with the rapidly increasing age of their populations, to the completely different problems faced by many developing countries. The dysfunctional health care systems of some of the latter often result from a lack of the basic necessities of hygiene and public health. In such situations, even inexpensive and well-tried approaches to medical care may not be available, reproductive health and perinatal care may be non-existent, and the basic amenities of clean water and adequate food may not be available.

These problems are highlighted by an analysis of over 11 million deaths due to infectious diseases in 1998 in which it was calculated that more than 3 million were due to diseases for which effective vaccines or other means of prevention are available (Widdus, 2001) (Box 4.1). Without a functioning health care system in place, with associated investment in health education, any benefits that result from genomics research will be irrelevant. These themes are considered in more detail in Section 7.

Throughout the consultations which preceded this Report, these complex issues concerning the discrepancies in standards of health care

Box 4.1   ANALYSIS OF DEATHS FROM INFECTIOUS DISEASES (1998)

Causes	Deaths
No satisfactory vaccine available when data compiled	
AIDS	2,285,000
Tuberculosis	1,498,000
Malaria	1,110,000
Pneumococcus	1,110,000
Rotavirus	800,000
Shigellosis	600,000
Enterotoxigenic *E. coli*	500,000
Respiratory syncytial virus	160,000
Schistosomiasis	150,000
Leishmaniasis	42,000
Trypanosomiasis	40,000
Chagas Disease	17,000
Dengue	15,000
Leprosy	2,000
Subtotal	*8,319,000*
Satisfactory vaccine available	
Hepatitis B	1,000,000
Measles	888,000
Haemophilus influenzae type B	500,000
Tetanus	410,000
Pertussis	346,000
Cholera	120,000
Diphtheria	5,000
Japanese encephalitis	3,000
Poliomyelitis	2,000
Subtotal	*3,274,000*
Grand Total	**11,593,000**

Source Widdus (2001).

throughout the world were continually stressed. Clearly, advances in genomics for global health care will have to be assessed with respect to their relative value in the practice and delivery of health care compared with the costs and efficacy of current approaches to public health, disease control, and the provision of basic preventive medicine and medical care.

4.2   WHEN WILL THE MEDICAL PROMISES OF GENOMICS BE FULFILLED?

Although the brief outline of the potential medical applications of genomics in Section 3 suggests that they will lead to major advances in clinical practice, it is difficult at the moment to predict the time-scale involved. Undoubtedly, an over-optimistic picture has emerged during the period of postgenome excitement (Burn et al., 2001). This has stemmed in part from a lack of appreciation of the complexity of many of the common killers of the developed world and those which will affect every country as it goes through the demographic transition. Furthermore, some scientists have tended to over emphasize the immediate medical importance of their work to the media or granting agencies, and companies have sometimes presented exaggerated claims, presumably to encourage their shareholders.

Some medical applications of the genome projects are, however, already with us. The diagnosis, prevention and, to some extent, management of monogenic disease was well advanced before the completion of the Human Genome Project. As well as providing new approaches to genetic counselling and the control of these diseases, information derived from work in genomics has pointed the way to learning more about the underlying causes of some common intractable diseases such as heart disease, hypertension and cancer.

Sufficient progress is being made in many different research programmes to suggest that within the next few years advances in technology which have followed the pathogen genome project will generate new vaccines and therapeutic agents. Similarly, there seems little doubt that there will be a steady flow of new diagnostic agents covering every aspect of communicable disease.

The time-scale for progress in the prevention and management of cancer is much less clear. It is likely that there will be a steady flow of new diagnostic approaches and tests for the identification of individuals at greater risk or for the early detection of different cancers, and that the further exploration of the patterns of oncogene mutations together with the increasing use of expression analyses will lead to the better classification of tumours, relating genotype to prognosis and, hopefully, to more logical forms of management. But because of the increasing evidence about the individuality of the genotypes of different cancers, it would be unwise to expect any single major development in treatment which will have applications right across the cancer field. Undoubtedly there will be surprises, the apparent specificity of the recently developed tyrosine kinase inhibitor for example, though even in this case drug resistance due to subtle changes in the abnormal kinase appeared quite soon. However, we know enough already to be confident that important progress will be made.

It is when we come to the possible fruits of the genetic analysis of the other common causes of mortality and morbidity in developed countries and those that are going through the demographic transition that we enter an area of real uncertainty. There are still considerable methodological and statistical problems to be overcome before it will be possible to carry out the proposed population analyses relating disease phenotypes to genetic markers (Altmuller et al., 2001; Roos, 2001). Information from the genome and related projects has provided a plethora of markers, but the planned association and linkage studies are fraught with uncertainties. Also, because of the relatively low level of heritability of many of these disorders, the likelihood that many genes will be involved, and problems of heterogeneity of disease phenotypes, it is very difficult to predict when information of this type will become of genuine value for predictive genetics and public health application. It is much more likely that at least some of this work will yield valuable clues to pathophysiological mechanisms and that this will be of more immediate value to the pharmaceutical industry in developing new therapeutic agents directed at specific gene products than for predictive genetics. It is possible that genetic profiling for susceptibility to common disease may, in the distant future, become part of programmes to focus public-health measures on high-risk groups, but many uncertainties remain (Weatherall, 1999; Wilkie, 2001).

It also seems likely that similar complexities will be encountered in attempts to develop pharmacogenomics to a level at which it is of genuine value in clinical practice. Even if the predicted rapid advances in this field come to fruition, and it is possible to develop genetic profiles of an individual patient's response to batteries of common drugs, the provision of the technology required for the primary care sector will present major organizational and financial problems. Also, will doctors use this information? It has been known for nearly 40 years that the metabolism of isoniazid, an important antituberculosis agent, varies widely due to easily identified variability in the function of a single-gene, and that this phenomenon is associated with a different pattern of therapeutic efficiency and side-effects, yet this information has rarely been used in clinical practice. Certainly, before pharmacogenomic programmes are introduced, careful pilot studies will have to be carried out to assess their efficacy and cost-effectiveness, together with programmes for the education of clinicians in the potential importance of this field.

There has been steady progress towards somatic-cell gene therapy, although there are still formidable problems to be overcome in obtaining long-term, high-level expression of inserted genes. For this reason it seems likely that the first important clinical applications will be for short-term objectives involving disease control, for example, the inhibition of tumour-cell proliferation or the unblocking of diseased arteries.

Similarly, it is difficult to predict when the results of research on embryonic stem cells for organ and tissue therapy will become relevant to clinical practice. There is widespread difference of opinion among countries about the ethical issues involved in the research on early embryos which will be required to move this field forward. Also, for research in this field which is confined to the private sector it is often very difficult to establish to what extent genuine progress is being made. Unless these ethical and organizational problems are resolved by strong international leadership, it is difficult to determine how rapidly the field will progress.

In short, for many potential areas of clinical application of the genome project there are still major concerns about the current state of the technology required and about whether at least some of the claims can be realized, and if so, when. However, enough progress has already been made in several areas of research in this rapidly moving and unpredictable field to suggest that the time has come to plan how this new technology and its potential clinical advances can be distributed among the world's population. The uncertainties in this field are not about whether the technology has the capacity to improve the health of the nations; some of the technological developments are already of proven value and should be applied now. What is not clear is how long it will take to reach its full potential, and how extensive (and expensive) that potential will be.

4.3 MAINTAINING THE BALANCE OF RESEARCH PLANNING AND HEALTH CARE

At the consultations that preceded this Report, it was stressed that there are widespread concerns among the international biomedical community and those who plan and administer health services that the hyperbole that has been generated by the genome projects and their aftermath will divert a disproportionate amount of funding into the field at the expense of more conventional and well-tried approaches to preventive medicine and clinical care. In many countries, concerns are also being raised about the apparent reduction in funding for research in community medicine, public health, primary care, epidemiology and clinical investigation compared with the huge expenditure on genomics.

It is important to put these fears into perspective. It is now over 20 years since the pharmaceutical industry produced a completely new antibiotic and, globally, communicable diseases remain major killers. New infective organisms, and new strains of existing pathogens which are resistant to all forms of treatment, are continually emerging. It is essential therefore that the completely new approach offered by the pathogen genome project is used to its full advantage. Similarly, the major reason for the escalation of the costs of health care in all the more developed countries is an inability to prevent and treat the major chronic illnesses of middle and old age. The same problems are already beginning to affect developing countries as they go through the demographic transition. Through the ingenuity of the pharmaceutical industry and clinical scientists, remarkable advances have been made in the symptomatic management of these diseases, but this high-technology, "patch-up" medicine is becoming increasingly expensive. The developed countries face a major financial and health-care crisis if this situation is allowed to continue.

In the period of uncertainty during which we are unclear about the level of the impact that work in the post-genome period will have on medical practice, it is important that international health agencies use their powers of advocacy to help governments ensure that a balance is maintained between research in public health, epidemiology, and clinical investigation compared to basic-science driven investigations in genomics and their applications. The vital role for WHO in this regard is considered in Section 10.

It is also essential to emphasize that none of the fruits of genomics research will take the place of the fundamental tenets of good clinical practice; it is particularly important to acknowledge this in the field of medical education. The traditional skills of history taking, careful clinical examination and the most economical use of simple laboratory and other ancillary investigations will remain the major approaches to diagnosis, treatment and the good pastoral care which is required increasingly in medical practice. At a time when medical care is coming under heavy criticism in many countries for its apparent lack of humanity and management of patients in a holistic manner, it is vital that this message is understood, as well as the importance of maintaining a balance between clinical and basic research, by those who are responsible for the provision of medical education and patient care.

4.4   WILL THE MEDICAL APPLICATIONS OF GENOME RESEARCH BE AFFORDABLE?

Because of the rising costs of medical care there is widespread anxiety that the developments that may stem from genomics research will be yet another example of an expensive high-technology practice to add to already over-stretched health economies. Can any country, regardless of its approach to the provision of health care, cope with the introduction of yet another extremely costly series of medical advances? Also, most relevant to this Report, will this new field simply widen the gap in the provision of care between the different countries of the world?

It is beyond the scope of this Report to consider the issues of the provision and distribution of the funding required to underpin the research and development of the biomedical advances that may stem from genomics. These important issues have been the subject of a recent report by the Commission on Macroeconomics and Health (2001). Among the Commission's recommendations for increasing expenditure on research and development is the suggestion that US$ 1.5 billion is funded through a new central organization, the Global Health Research Fund, support that would be directed at basic biomedical and health research and which would be available, through peer-reviewed application, to every country. A second US$ 1.5 billion should be made available for institutions which are working on new vaccine and drug development for HIV/AIDS, tuberculosis and malaria. Although the mechanisms for the distribution of increased funding along these lines will require further work, without a major international incentive of this kind, and input from the richer nations, it is difficult to see how the biomedical potential of genomics for health will be realized, particularly in the developing countries.

Although it is clear that genomics research is already consuming large amounts of biomedical research funding (see Section 7), and because up to now it has yielded so few applications for the clinic, it is much too early to determine the costs of the potential benefits of this field. Interestingly, preliminary cost-benefit analyses for the development of DNA-based control programmes for the haemoglobin disorders, or for the use of DNA diagnostics for some communicable diseases, suggest that the introduction of this technology will be cost-effective (WHO, 1994; Harris and Tanner, 2000). Each new set of screening or diagnostic procedures will have to be subjected to pilot studies to assess their cost-effectiveness before they are introduced into clinical practice. But because of the greater ease and precision of many forms of DNA diagnostics compared with other approaches, it seems likely that they will slowly become a valuable and cost-effective addition to programmes for disease diagnosis and control.

The position regarding the development of therapeutic agents and vaccines is far less clear. Companies will have to recoup the enormous expenditure on research and development that will be required to take advantage of the genomics approach to drug and vaccine design. Particularly because much of the technology is new and unexplored, the initial costs of these products may be very high. On the other hand, because of the potential for faster and more efficient ways of identifying therapeutic agents and vaccine candidates, and the possibility that they could offer more definitive control or cure of intractable diseases, in the longer-term costs could well fall. It is simply too early to be able to make any sensible predictions.

The problems involved in trying to ensure that the costs of advances in genomics for health care do not increase the inequality of health provision between nations are discussed in Sections 5 and 7.

Due to these uncertainties about the costs of the fruits of genomic research, Section 5 argues for a slow and incremental introduction of DNA technology into the developing countries. This should be based on those technologies which have already been shown to be cost-effective, or those in which it would be relatively easy to find out whether this is the case by the use of small pilot studies.

4.5   SUMMARY

In recognition of the fact that it is a new and rapidly evolving branch of science, the future role of genomics for the provision of health care is far from clear. However, it does offer the long-term possibility of providing new approaches to the prevention and management of many intractable diseases. Hence it is important to prepare society for the complexities of this new field, to ensure that its benefits are distributed fairly among the countries of the world, and that the well-tried and more conventional approaches to medical research and practice are not neglected while the medical potential of genomics is being explored.

5. The Potential of Genomics for the Health of the Developing Countries

5.1   Introduction

So far the clinical applications of genomics and molecular medicine have been very limited, even in the developed countries in which this work has been pursued. This is not surprising; the discovery of the organism that causes tuberculosis was announced in 1881 and yet it was not until 70 years later that streptomycin was developed. There is always a lag between major developments in the research laboratory and their full application in the clinic. But, just as in the case of tuberculosis at the turn of the century, much is learnt which is of benefit to patients in the interim. The technological developments that will result from genomics and molecular medicine will undoubtedly facilitate many of the areas of research that have been outlined in previous sections, with a steady pipeline of important medical applications before they come to their full fruition for health care. Many of these advances will have direct application to health care in developing countries.

Hence in discussing the role of molecular medicine and genomics for improving the health of the developing countries, it is helpful to consider the following questions:

1. Which areas of human and pathogen genomics have reached the stage of development at which they have direct application in the clinic or the field, which of these clinical advances are most germane to the needs of the developing countries, how can the DNA technology that underpins them be most effectively developed in these countries, and

how can this be achieved without a major increase in expenditure on health care?

2. In the many areas of potential medical application of the fruits of genomics which still require extensive research and development before they are of clinical value, to what extent should developing countries become involved in the work that is required? To what extent are the medical research and biotechnology capabilities of some of these countries sufficiently advanced already for developing networks between them to facilitate this research?

3. Since there are still major uncertainties about the relative roles of academia and industry in pursuing post-genomic research, and particularly its practical applications, what will be the most effective way of developing partnerships between the developed and developing countries so that the medical applications of this new field can be made available to humankind in general? Are there models of collaborations of this kind in existence already on which to build for the future?

5.2   EXAMPLES OF WHAT IS FEASIBLE NOW

Currently, in some developed countries, recombinant DNA technology is firmly established in clinical genetics, where it is being used widely for genetic counselling, prenatal diagnosis, and, to a limited degree, for population screening. The development of technologies based on PCR, an ingenious way of rapidly amplifying particular DNA sequences, is playing a small but steadily increasing role in diagnostic genetics, prognostic pathology, microbiology and virology. There are relatively few recombinant therapeutic agents and vaccines available, but, as described earlier, many promising leads are being followed up. Somatic-cell gene therapy still has very limited applications.

However, taking these limited clinical applications together with extensive consultation on health priorities with member countries, it is clear that there are some important areas of health provision based on DNA technology which could be developed in many countries without delay. Furthermore, there are major advantages in moving quickly in this direction. By providing the training and technology to pursue what is currently feasible and already of importance in health care, it will be possible to establish the technological base on which to benefit from the advances which will come from the genome projects as they evolve in the future.

The examples of the immediate value of transferring recombinant DNA technology to the developing world which follow are all based on the priorities for health care which were defined during the consultations that preceded this Report, and are all compatible with the concept of the evolution of a technological base for future development.

5.2.1 THE INHERITED DISORDERS OF HAEMOGLOBIN.

The sickle-cell diseases and the thalassaemias are the commonest monogenic diseases in the world and, as described earlier (Section 3.2), are imposing an increasing drain on health resources, particularly as countries go through the demographic transition. These diseases are nearly all Mendelian recessive conditions; affected children (homozygotes) receive the gene for these conditions from each of their symptomless (carrier) parents.

The control and management of these disorders is now well-established in some developed countries but thousands of children are dying from these conditions in poorer parts of the world. Furthermore, because these are genetic disorders and there is no definitive cure for any of them, and this is likely to be the case for the foreseeable future, they pose a particularly difficult problem; unlike communicable disease, they require a lifetime of medical treatment. For example, a recent collaborative study between Indonesian researchers and those from developed countries on the gene frequency for thalassaemia in Indonesia predicts that about 1.25 to 1.5 million units of blood per year will be required to treat the thalassaemic population in the near future (de Silva et al., 2000). Many countries are adding thousands of new patients with these diseases to their medical care programmes each year, yet the technology is now well advanced for screening, counselling and prenatal detection, and cost-effective programmes for disease control in the Mediterranean islands and elsewhere are well-established (Box 5.1). When considering technology transfer for the control of these diseases it is important to distinguish the requirements for the thalassaemias from those for the sickle-cell disorders.

Hundreds of different mutations that give rise to the thalassaemias have been identified and simple and cheap techniques have been developed for carrier detection. Because the severe forms of disease require lifelong transfusion and expensive drugs for removing iron that accumulates in multitransfused children, and because of the increasing costs of screening donated blood for pathogens, many countries have opted for prenatal screening and, if parents find it acceptable, prenatal diagnosis and termi-

---

Box 5.1   POPULATION CONTROL OF COMMON DISORDERS OF HAEMOGLOBIN

Essential steps for the establishment clinical genetic services for the control of thalassemias and sickle-cell diseases

1. Population survey to assess gene frequency.

2. Community education programme and counselling.

3. Set up a reference laboratory, community clinics and a screening programme.

4. Define patterns of screening
   General: School leavers or other population groups.
   Sickle cell diseases: Neonatal screening for prophylactic treatment, prenatal screening if prenatal diagnosis is intended.
   For thalassemia: Prenatal screening if prenatal diagnosis is intended

5. Screening
   Sickle cell diseases: Sickle test
   α or β thalassemia: Red-cell indices (size and volume)

6. Confirmatory tests
   Sickle cell diseases: Haemoglobin electrophoresis
   β thalassemia: HbA_2 estimation. Gene analysis[*]
   α thalassemia: Exclusion by normal HbA_2 estimation. Gene analysis[**]

7. Further Actions
   Family study
   Genetic counselling
   Decision about prenatal diagnosis if both parents are carriers
   Early discussion of management issues for affected babies

[*] Gene analysis required for prenatal diagnosis or for counselling regarding severity.

[**] α thalassemia can only be diagnosed with certainty by DNA analysis.

---

nation of pregnancy if the fetus is affected. Even where termination is not currently acceptable it is clear that objections based on religious and cultural beliefs are changing. To establish thalassaemia control programmes, one or two central diagnostic laboratories with the ability to analyse haemoglobin and to identify mutations by DNA technology are required, together with a network of peripheral clinics with staff trained in counselling and simple and cheap screening methods. These relatively straightforward requirements, supported by a major national education programme, are the foundations on which thalassaemia control has been established in many countries (Box 5.1).

Currently, the state of development of the expertise required to run national control programmes for thalassaemia varies widely. It is well-established in the USA, and in European and Mediterranean countries, and in some parts of the Middle East and the Indian subcontinent. In Asia the technology is available in Thailand, where control programmes are being established, and a start has been made in Indonesia. But there are many countries in which the control and management of thalassaemia are not yet established. In many of those in which programmes are underway they have evolved in collaboration with developed countries and their success is a model on which programmes can be developed in the future. Furthermore, because there is expertise already in many regions, the possibilities for developing local networks are considerable.

The problems posed by sickle-cell anaemia are different from those associated with thalassaemia. This disease is particularly common in sub-Saharan Africa, where it has been estimated that there may be up to 300,000 affected babies born each year. It also occurs sporadically in some Mediterranean populations and at particularly high frequencies in some of the oasis populations of the Middle East and in parts of India. Unlike the case of the severe forms of thalassaemia, children with sickle cell anemia do not usually require lifelong transfusion but they are prone to painful episodes of bone pain and more serious complications arising from sequestration of sickle cells in the spleen, lungs or liver. The commonest cause of death is infection, to which these children are particularly prone.

In the African-American populations of North America and in the Caribbean, neonatal screening programmes and the administration of oral penicillin has resulted in a marked reduction in the mortality of sickle-cell anaemia in childhood, but because of its variable course prenatal detection and prenatal diagnosis have not been practised widely except in a few European countries. The effects of the demographic transition on the frequency of symptomatic patients with sickle-cell anaemia is very similar to that for thalassaemia. In rural regions of sub-Saharan Africa it is very likely that the majority of babies and young children with sickle cell anaemia die early in life, mainly from infection which may lead to profound anaemia. As evidenced by the urbanized populations of Africa, many more children with this condition are surviving and the same phenomena is being observed throughout the Middle East and in India.

Just as in the case of thalassaemia, a great deal could be done to improve the lot of patients with sickle cell anaemia in developing countries. Although DNA technology is valuable for identifying the complex interactions of the sickle cell gene with different forms of thalassaemia and other haemoglobin variants, countries with a high frequency of the sickle cell gene would only need one central reference laboratory in which this technology is available. The development of peripheral screening clinics, directed particularly at neonatal screening, and the availability of oral penicillin prophylaxis, would have a major effect on survival of patients with the sickle cell disorders in Africa and throughout the Middle East and India. The screening techniques are cheap and simple but need to be supported by a major education programme for local clinicians in the management of the complications of the disease, which occur throughout the lives of patients with this condition. But most importantly, no screening programme should be established until adequate counselling and public education programmes are in place.

There is therefore abundant evidence that the inherited anaemias could be controlled and that the main problems at the moment are a lack of awareness of their importance, lack of organization, and limited availability of relatively simple diagnostic procedures. The development of centres with expertise in screening, DNA diagnosis, education, counselling and management of these conditions would provide the basis on which clinical genetics services could evolve in many developing countries. In the thalassaemia field many countries already have expertise in the diagnosis and prevention of the disease, and others are just starting to evolve programmes of this type. In the case of the sickle-cell disorders there are a few centres in the Caribbean, India and the Middle East with the expertise required to develop and establish community prevention programmes. Similarly, there are centres in Ghana, Kenya, Nigeria and other countries where this knowledge is available. Thus, here again there is a major opportunity for developing regional networks between different countries to develop and establish control programmes.

The establishment of prenatal diagnosis programmes for thalassaemia is a valuable model of cooperation between the developed and developing countries which, when combined with local networking, could provide the expertise to result in a major reduction in the increasing public health burden posed by the haemoglobin disorders.

5.2.2   GENETIC RESISTANCE TO COMMUNICABLE DISEASE

Work carried out over recent years is providing increasing evidence that a varying proportion of many different populations have genetically determined resistance to important infectious diseases, including malaria, tuberculosis and HIV/AIDS (Box 5.2). Furthermore, careful case control studies have started to quantify these effects and they are not trivial (Cooke and Hill, 2001).

In the case of malaria, for example, at least in certain African populations, the sickle-cell trait affords over 80% protection against the severe

Box 5.2   EXAMPLES OF HUMAN GENES INVOLVED IN VARYING SUSCEPTIBILITY TO COMMUNICABLE DISEASE

Disease	Genes influencing susceptibility
Malaria	α-globin; β-globin; Duffy chemokine receptor; G6PD; Blood group O; Erythrocyte band 3; HLA-B; HLA-DR; TNF; ICAM-1; Spectrin; Glycophorin A; Glycophorin B; CD36
Tuberculosis	HLA-A; HLA-DR; SLC11A1; VDR; IFNγR1
HIV/AIDS	CCR5; CCR2; IL-10
Leprosy	HLA-DR
Hepatitis-B	HLA-DR; IL-10
Acute bacterial infection	MBL-2; FCγRII-R; Sec 2

G6PD: glucose-6-phosphate deficiency

TNF: tumour necrosis factor

ICAM: intercellular adhesion network

SLC11A1: solute carrier family 11, member 1

VRD: vitamin D receptor

CCR-5: chemokine receptor 5

IL-10: interleukin 10

IFNγR1: interferon-γ receptor-1

MBL: mannose binding lectin

FCgRII-R: receptor for constant region of immunoglobulin

Sec: secretor of blood group substance

complications of *Plasmodium falciparum* malaria, particularly cerebral malaria and severe anaemia; and α thalassaemia offers 60% protection against these complications in Papua New Guinea. Remarkably, the form of inherited ovalocytosis (oval red blood cells) that is common in Melanesia offers complete protection against cerebral malaria. These genetic conditions are common, ranging from up to 20% or more for the sickle cell trait in some African countries to 10–80% for α thalassaemia in many tropical populations (Weatherall and Clegg, 2001). There are many other genetic variants involved in malaria resistance (Box 5.2) and it is not yet known to what extent their protective effect may be additive within a particular population.

Clearly, if malaria vaccine trials are carried out in populations in tropical developing countries, and particularly if the end result is amelioration rather than total protection, it will be vital to know ahead of time if a considerable proportion of the population is relatively resistant to the disease already. This information should be obtained before the trial starts or even at the planning stages. Since some programmes of this type will require control (untreated) populations, it will also be important to determine whether the local resistance polymorphisms are equally represented among them and the population being treated. The technology required to determine the frequency of these polymorphisms varies in sophistication. For example, it involves only a simple blood test for sickling, whereas the identification of many polymorphisms requires relatively simple DNA technology, very similar to that outlined in the previous section for the identification of the haemoglobin variants. Since the frequency of these different polymorphisms varies enormously from country to country, it will be necessary for it to be determined for each individual population under investigation.

5.2.3   THE INTRODUCTION OF DNA DIAGNOSTICS FOR COMMUNICABLE DISEASE

The place of DNA diagnostics in the management and control of communicable disease is not yet certain and is currently the subject of widespread debate and controversy. While it is clear that DNA diagnostics will not replace many of the well-tried methods of culture and serology, they are turning out to be of considerable value for the identification of organisms which are difficult or impossible to culture and for assessing the level of activity of chronic viral infections. For example, they are of considerable value in monitoring the activity level of infection and potential need for treatment in patients with hepatitis C infections and in the diagnosis of some forms of viral meningitis, particularly those due to herpes simplex infections.

Work in Latin America has suggested that the diagnosis of dengue fever and leishmaniasis has been improved by the use of PCR and that this technique is proving more rapid, sensitive, and versatile, and, most importantly, less costly than current methods for the detection of a wide range of pathogenic organisms (Box 5.3). These encouraging observations suggest that similar pilot studies should be established in other developing countries to assess the reliability and cost-effectiveness of DNA diagnostics for pathogens that are common in their populations (Harris et al., 1993; Harris and Tanner, 2000).

5.2.4   DRUG-RESISTANT ORGANISMS

While there is no doubt that the scope of DNA diagnostics for the identification of organisms which are difficult to isolate or culture will increase,

Box 5.3   Adaptation and Transfer of Molecular Techniques for Application to Public Health Programmes in Developing Countries

The work of Eva Harris and her colleagues at the Sustainable Sciences Institute (SSI, San Francisco, CA, USA) has demonstrated how the techniques of modern molecular biology may be readily transferred and adapted to local conditions in developing countries and harnessed to address local priorities for improving public health.

Professor Harris and her collaborators initiated the Applied Molecular Biology/ Appropriate Technology Transfer (AMB/ATT) programme in the early 1990s — multi-stage on-site training workshops that introduced the techniques of molecular biology, epidemiology and scientific writing to researchers in developing Latin American countries, in order to enhance their capacity to initiate independent research. The workshops focused on the adaptation of molecular biomedical techniques to local research priorities and conditions. AMB/ATT aimed to help the countries build the scientific capability to undertake locally relevant research — an essential prerequisite for the development of public health programmes. It addressed some of the major barriers faced — including limited access to technologies, scientific isolation, a lack of information and the absence of technical training programmes.

In 1998, Professor Harris and her collaborators established the Sustainable Sciences Institute (SSI), a not-for-profit non-governmental organization to further these technology transfer programmes. SSI has continued the AMB/ATT programmes. Workshops have been held in Nicaragua, Ecuador, Guatemala, Bolivia, Cuba, Venezuela, Paraguay and the USA and have to date trained over 400 scientists and health professionals in 19 developing countries, sparking collaborative projects, locally funded proposals and scientific publications.

In addition, SSI has developed a small grants programme to provide research support to scientists in developing countries, a database of voluntary consultants offering expert advice for technology transfer activities, and a material aid programme to facilitate the transfer of scientific equipment and supplies from biotech companies and university laboratories in developed countries to laboratories in developing countries. Above all, the SSI is committed to fostering the long-term stable partnerships between technology donors and recipients upon which successful technology transfer depends, and supporting the ongoing guidance that recipients require.

These programmes have demonstrated conclusively that molecular technologies can be adapted to local conditions and disease priorities in developing countries to be more rapid, versatile and sensitive than alternative methods. Furthermore, they can be cost-effective in low-budget situations. It has been shown for example that PCR protocols can be introduced at as little as one-hundredth of the cost of commercially-available assays through a myriad of inventive approaches including simplification of protocols, bulk preparation of reagents from crude ingredients, and recycling.

Through holding training workshops on-site, local scientists begin to learn how the technologies may be adapted to local conditions. In many cases, these scientists have then used their ingenuity to refine the technologies further. Importantly, the knowledge based approach that presents both the advantages and limitations of new technologies allows local scientists to make a well-informed decision about their utility on a case-by-case basis.

The adoption of the technologies introduced through these workshops has already been implemented to enhance public health programmes in Latin America. PCR has been

Box 5.3 (CONTINUED)

adopted as a routine diagnostic procedure for leishmaniasis by the Nicaraguan Ministry of Health, having proved to be simpler and more sensitive than existing techniques. PCR has also improved detection methods for dengue in Nicaragua and Paraguay. It was used in 1995 to rule out dengue as the cause of an outbreak of hemorrhagic fever in northern Nicaragua, which led to the identification of leptospirosis as the culprit and its recognition worldwide as a major emerging disease. In Paraguay, timely use of recently-implemented molecular typing methods enabled containment of a dengue outbreak in the capital Asunción in 2001.

References

1. Harris EM, Lopez J, Arevalo J, Bellatin A, Belli J, Moran, et al. (1993). Short courses on DNA detection and amplification for public health in Central and South America: the democratization of molecular biology. *Biochemical Education* 21:16–22.

2. Harris E (1996). Developing essential scientific capability in countries with limited resources. *Nature Medicine* 2: 737–739.

3. Harris E, Kadir N (1998). *A Low-Cost Approach to PCR : Appropriate Transfer of Biomolecular Techniques* New York, Oxford University Press

4. Harris E, Tanner M (2000). Health technology transfer. *British Medical Journal,* 321:817–820.

5. The Sustainable Sciences Institute (Website http://www.sslink.org).

there is a more immediate application of this technology which may be of considerable economic importance for many developing countries.

There have already been successes in defining some of the genes that are responsible for drug resistance in important pathogens, including those responsible for tuberculosis, HIV/AIDS and malaria. For example, mutations in the chloroquine resistance transporter of *Plasmodium falciparum*, encoded by the gene *pfcrt*, confer chloroquine resistance in laboratory strains of the parasite. Recent studies in Mali showed that there is a stable relationship between rates of the chloroquine-resistant genotype and *in-vivo* chloroquine resistance at sites where there are different population sizes, ethnic compositions and levels of drug resistance and malaria transmission (Djimdé et al., 2001). This approach appears to have the potential to be of considerable value for public health surveillance of antimalarial resistance and may permit comprehensive mapping of resistance at country and regional levels without the need to carry out numerous repeated longitudinal efficacy studies, particularly in central and west Africa where chloroquine use remains widespread.

The increasing ability to monitor rapidly large samples of organisms for drug resistance, and to maintain regular surveillance of the emergence of resistant strains, is likely to be an important addition to the public health measures directed at the control of many important pathogens. Indeed, the epidemiological technology which is almost certain to be derived from the pathogen genome project will undoubtedly play a major role in disease prevention in the future.

A great deal more research is still required to assess the relative roles of DNA technology and conventional methods for assessing drug resistance, and to assess the relationship between resistance markers and lack of clinical response. Work of this kind has to be carried out in the countries in which these pathogens occur frequently.

Since the pattern of emergence of drug resistant pathogens varies widely between different countries it will be extremely important for every region of the developing world to pursue this research and to have access to this technology and, where this is not possible, to develop it itself. As information from the pathogen genome project becomes available, it should be possible for countries to develop similar approaches to their own particular pathogens. Again, the DNA technology involved is relatively simple and easily transferable.

5.2.5 PHARMACOGENOMICS

There is increasing evidence that individual variation among individuals in drug response may have important implications for the control of important communicable diseases in the developing countries. For example, recent studies have shown that the frequency of a particular polymorphism for the gene *MDR1* is much more common in West African and African American populations than in those of European or Japanese background (Schaeffeler et al., 2001). This gene regulates the expression of P-glycoprotein which is important in defence mechanisms against potentially toxic agents ingested in the diet. It has been suggested that this variant of the *MDR1* gene is common in Africa because it has offered a selective advantage against gastrointestinal-tract infections. However, it appears that this gene reduces the efficacy of drugs such as protease inhibitors and related agents which are now widely used for the treatment of HIV-1 infections.

Currently, there is very little evidence about the practical implications of individual variation in drug response of this kind, particularly regarding its effect on the efficacy of the treatment of conditions like HIV/AIDS. At a time when major efforts are being made to provide adequate supplies of drugs for the treatment of HIV infections in the developing countries, and attempts are being made to overcome the difficulties of delivering them to the patients that need them, it is important that pilot studies to determine the effect of genetic variation in drug response are incorporated into these programmes. If genetic variation of this type has an important effect on the outcome of treatment, it will have major clinical and financial implications for the management of common communicable diseases.

5.2.6 NON-COMMUNICABLE DISEASE

As described in earlier sections, the application of molecular genetics and the fruits of the Human Genome Project have not yet had much direct application for the prevention and care of the common causes of chronic ill-health in developed countries, particularly heart disease, stroke, diabetes and cancer. However hopes for the future are pinned on genomics leading to a better understanding of their pathogenesis and hence the development of completely new approaches to prevention and therapy.

Given the more pressing needs of the developing countries with respect to the provision of the basics of adequate health care, together with the enormous problems posed by communicable disease, it is, at first sight, not obvious why they should even be considering utilizing their limited facilities for research and development towards these less-pressing health problems. There is, however, increasing evidence that these diseases are already presenting important challenges in many countries that are undergoing the demographic transition (Alberti, 2001). Indeed, recent figures indicate that almost twice as many people die from these conditions in the developing than the developed countries.

A prime example is the world epidemic of insulin-resistant (type 2) diabetes, which is an extremely important risk factor for vascular disease. Although accurate epidemiological data are difficult to obtain, it appears that this disease is reaching frequencies of between 20% and 70% in many populations and that the global figure of affected people will rise from the current figure of 150 million to 300 million by 2025 (Zimmet et al., 2001). At the same time, hypertension and vascular disease are rapidly increasing problems in various African, Asian and Caribbean countries. Indeed, the picture that is emerging is that many of the developing countries that are struggling to improve basic standards of nutrition and hygiene, and that are attempting to control the problems of communicable disease, are then finding themselves facing an unusually high frequency of these major causes of morbidity and mortality in adult life (Unwin et al., 2001).

The reasons for the global epidemic of type 2 diabetes are not yet understood and are the subject of one of the most intense scientific debates in the biomedical research field. Monogenic forms of the diseases are rare, accounting for only 2 to 3% of cases. However, twin studies, though they have given rather inconsistent results, have suggested that there is a strong genetic component to this condition. Evolutionary biologists have suggested that it may reflect the selection of what is called a "thrifty genotype" which confers the ability in the distant past to undergo long periods of dietary privation, a genetic make-up which is now totally unsuited to the high-energy diets of the developed countries. On the other hand, more recent epidemiological research has pointed to the possible importance of low birth weight in establishing a series of metabolic pathways which may be associated with obesity, insulin resistance and the development of type 2 diabetes in later life.

It seems likely, therefore, that the syndrome of obesity and type 2 diabetes reflects the action of a number of different genes, combined with a changing environment. In other words, they reflect a response to environmental change and altered risk factors which may vary between different populations depending on their genetic make-up. If some of the genetic polymorphisms involved are quite ancient, it is likely that the pathogenesis of this disease may vary considerably among different human populations. Furthermore, there may well be populations which, because of their relatively small number of founders, are particularly valuable for trying to dissect the genetic component.

Given the urgency of this problem, and the mutual benefit for both the developed and developing countries in determining how to control type 2 diabetes, and because of the likely genetic heterogeneity and variability of other environmental factors involved, this seems an ideal disease in which to pursue an international partnership in research and development. There are already a number of collaborative programmes between universities and research institutes in developed and developing countries in this field, and at least some companies in developed countries are initiating international research programmes, partly because they have appreciated the value of studying populations with a very high frequency of this condition. But unless these genome-related studies are backed up with equally competent epidemiological studies, this field is unlikely to move forward as quickly as it could.

There is a major need for international leadership in the co-ordination of these studies, particularly with respect to defining agreed phenotypes and in distinguishing between the relative roles of genes and the environment in the development of diabetes and insulin resistance in different populations. There are already a number of university-based and industrial groups in Europe and the USA who have the background and expertise in this field, and which could provide an international base for development of this kind. Some of them already have experience with partnerships in the developing countries and with further international leadership by international organizations, this programme could be developed very quickly.

As it is becoming increasingly common, type 2 diabetes has been discussed as a model for the importance of evolving developed-developing country partnerships for establishing research programmes for the study of non-communicable disease in the developing countries. However, other conditions which are becoming more prevalent in these populations are also amenable to the same approach. For example, cardiac disease and hypertension is particularly common in some populations and it is estimated that bipolar affective disorders will be the commonest cause of chronic ill-health globally by the year 2020.

It is important, however, to consider the role of genomics in the further study and control of these common disorders in the context of current public health efforts directed towards the same end. Conventional epidemiological studies have provided convincing evidence that type 2 diabetes and cardiovascular disease, together with many forms of cancer, are related to definable risk factors such as cigarette smoking, obesity, and a variety of dietary changes. Clearly, it is important that a high priority is given to public education leading to a reduction in these risk factors.

On the other hand, it is important to follow up the leads towards the possible elucidation of the basic causes of these conditions through the application of genomics because, however effective the more direct public health measures are, these conditions will continue to prove to be a major drain on health resources. Because of the likelihood that their basic causes vary between different populations, the development of more effective forms of control and treatment will require an understanding of the individual disease mechanisms involved.

5.3   THE DEVELOPMENT AND PROVISION OF SERVICES IN CLINICAL GENETICS AND DNA TECHNOLOGY

The examples of the control of the haemoglobin disorders and other applications of DNA technology discussed above (Section 5.2) could be extended to any genetic diseases which are common enough to constitute a major health burden. Furthermore, the requirements for controlling the haemoglobin disorders provide a model for the development of other genetic services. This will involve the training of a sufficient number of medical personnel to provide expertise in clinical genetics, including the new and increasingly important field of genetic epidemiology. It must also include the education and technical training of nurses and genetic counsellors who are well versed in the problems of genetic screening and the kind of educational information that is required for the development of community programmes of this type. This kind of specialized programme will have to be augmented by a much broader education of primary care clinicians who have to make the decision for or against referral to expert centres for genetic testing. Many of these issues are discussed in two WHO reports, *Community control of genetic and congenital disorders* (WHO, 1997) and *Primary health care approaches for prevention and control of congenital and genetic disorders* (WHO, 2000).

The principle of establishing centres with expertise in DNA diagnosis, as outlined for clinical genetics services, seems to provide the most effective way of introducing DNA technology into developing countries. There are already many examples of how this has been achieved in the case of the haemoglobin disorders. This approach to technology transfer has the great value of introducing a new field of expertise that can be seen to provide immediate health benefits to the community in a country which receives the technology. Furthermore, once there is a critical mass of facilities of this type, the technology can be easily transferred to other disciplines, the control of communicable disease and the study of other common health problems in particular communities, for example. Also, by appropriate local networking, other clinical specialities can start to introduce DNA technology into their own fields. Hence, there is a major role for WHO in helping to establish basic genetic services throughout the world.

5.4   GENOMICS FOR THE CONTROL OF COMMUNICABLE DISEASE: FUTURE DIRECTIONS

It is clear from the consultations which preceded this Report that the top priority for the development of medical benefits from genomics in many developing countries is for the improved control of communicable disease. As outlined in Section 2, genomics offers major opportunities for the development of new vaccines, diagnostics and therapeutic agents.

The biotechnology and pharmaceutical industries of developed countries, together with academia and support from the medical charities, are tackling some of the key communicable diseases, for example tuberculosis, HIV/AIDS and malaria, although the total expenditure on research and development for these conditions is only a small fraction of that spent on non-communicable disease (See Section 7). But there is far less research directed at important infectious diseases that are more localized in their distribution, for example dengue and melioidosis in parts of Asia and Chagas disease in South America.

Hence it will be important for individual countries to set their priorities for developing their own pathogen genome programmes. This would seem to be a good starting point for utilizing the extensive opportunities for drug design in general which are likely to stem from the human and pathogen genome projects. Although some of the research required will be carried out in academic and related institutions, reaping the full benefits will require early input from the commercial sector.

The current state of expertise in biotechnology outside developed countries varies widely across the world. Many countries, such as China, Cuba, India, Indonesia, Korea, Singapore, and Thailand, and some of those in South America have already developed considerable expertise in biotechnology. The examples of Brazil, China and India and the Asia-Pacific Region, which have each developed world-class capacity in many areas of genomics research, are highlighted in Boxes 5.4, 5.5, 5.6 and 5.7, respectively.

One of the major problems faced by developing countries is retaining their most talented scientists, who are often tempted by better working facilities and higher salaries in the developed countries. For example, it has been estimated that 30 000 PhD holders of African descent live and work outside their countries of origin, a figure that far exceeds the total working in Africa (Hassan, 2001). In China, this problem is being approached at least in part by the development of joint appointments, whereby some of their scientists spend part of their time in the developed countries. While this field is still developing, this type of approach, both between the industrial and university sectors, seems to be a possible way forward.

There are, however, major problems for many developing countries, particularly those of sub-Saharan Africa, which have not yet been able to evolve biotechnology capabilities within their less substantial, and in some cases non-existent pharmaceutical industries. The danger here is that these

Box 5.4   Brazil — Local Networking for Capacity Building in Genomics
The strategies adopted by Brazil over the last five years have propelled the country into the upper echelons of international genomics research. Its approach of building a national research network provides a valuable model for other countries. In 1997, the Sao Paulo state research funding foundation, FAPESP, made a strategic decision to initiate a major genomics research programme. It was decided that the first goal of this programme would be to sequence the genome of the bacterium, *Xylella fastidiosa*, a pathogen of citrus crops which is estimated to cost the Brazilian economy more than US$ 100 million each year in lost income.

Rather than building a single sequencing centre to undertake this work, FAPESP initiated a "virtual genomics institute," a network of approximately 200 researchers based at 30 laboratories throughout the state of Sao Paulo, supported by an initial budget of US$ 13 million. The five or six existing centres within this network with some expertise in genomics served as training hubs to pass on the techniques to other laboratories. The network had a defined management structure, and rapidly developed Internet systems to link and coordinate the participating centres. It became known as the Organization for Nucleotide Sequencing and Analysis (ONSA).

The network sequenced 90% of the three million base *Xylella* genome in less than one year, and published the complete sequence in *Nature* in July 2000. This remarkable achievement received considerable media attention both in Brazil and globally, demonstrating both to the international research community and the Brazilian public, that the country could play a world leading role in scientific research. Brazil is now an undisputed leader in plant pathogen genomics and has developed three further genome sequencing programmes for agriculturally-important pathogens and a *Xylella* functional genomics network.

A second major ONSA programme, the Cancer Genome Project was launched in March 1999, supported by US$ 10 million funding from FAPESP and the Ludwig Institute for Cancer Research. The aim of the project was to identify expressed sequence tags (ESTs) associated with various types of cancer, especially those of the stomach, head and neck which are particularly prevalent in Brazil. The project utilized the ORETES technique for isolating complementary DNAs through low stringency PCR which was pioneered at the Ludwig Institute in Brazil.

This project has been phenomenally successful — a week after the announcement of the *Xylella* sequence, the Cancer Project announced that it had mapped half a million ESTs. In October 2001, the group published in the *Proceedings of the National Academy of Sciences, USA* the identification of 700 000 sequence tags active in 24 normal and cancerous tissues. This work suggests that initial estimates of the total number of human genes might be too low. Brazil now ranks alongside the USA and the United Kingdom as a world leader in cancer genomics research and is developing strong collaborative links with the US National Cancer Institute.

Building on these achievements, FAPESP is expanding and diversifying ONSA's activities — launching a viral genetic discovery network, a schistosomiasis genome project and a project to characterize ESTs from sugar cane. It has also initiated a national structural genomics programme for high throughput protein structure determination.

Stimulated by the achievement of FAPESP, the Brazilian Ministry of Science and Technology in partnership with the National Council for Scientific and Technological Development (CNPQ) launched in late 2000 a distinct nationwide sequencing network including 25 sequencing laboratories distributed from the Amazon to the borders of

Box 5.4 (CONTINUED)

Uruguay. Despite the enormous distances involved this network has also been an outstanding success and is in the final stages of sequencing the relatively large bacterial genome of *Chromobacterium violaceum*, which is of significant biotechnological importance. A number of other local sequence networks are being financed by CNPQ to undertake a variety of projects of both agricultural and public health importance.

Brazil has developed world-leading genomics research capabilities in a remarkably short period of time. Sequencing networks in Brazil encompass over 70 laboratories, and now includes the entire country. Although, a number of major challenges remain, there is little doubt that other countries can learn much from its capacity building strategies.

References

1. Simpson AJG, Reinach FC, Arruda P, Abreu FA, Acencio M, Alvarenga R, et al. (2000). The genome sequence of the plant pathogen *Xylella fastidiosa*. *Nature* 406:151–157.

2. de Souza SJ, Camargo AA, Briones MRS, Costa FF, Nagai MA, Verjovski-Almeida S, et al. (2000). The identification of human chromosome 22 transcribed sequences with ORF expressed sequence tags. *Proceedings of the National Academy of Sciences, USA*, 97: 12690–12693.

3. Camargo AA, Samaia HPB, Dias-Neto E, Simão DF, Migotto IA, Briones MRS, et al. (2001). The contribution of 700,000 ORF sequence tags to the definition of the human transcriptome *Proceedings of the National Academy of Sciences, USA*, 98: 12103–12108.

4. Macilwain C, Neto RB (2000). A springboard to success. *Nature* 407:440–441

5. The Organization for Nucleotide and Sequence Analysis (ONSA) (Website http://watson.fapesp.br/genoma3.htm)

Box 5.5   CHINA — BUILDING A BASIS FOR POST-GENOMIC SCIENCE

Over recent years, the Chinese government has made a concerted drive to move China into the vanguard of genomics research. In early 1998, the Ministry of Science and Technology established the Chinese National Human Genome Centre (CHGC), based in Beijing and Shanghai, and the Beijing Institute of Genomics (BGI) as centres of excellence for genome sequencing and analysis. The establishment of these facilities enabled China to join the International Human Genome Sequencing Consortium in 1999. China played a key role in the project, taking responsibility for characterising 1% of the three billion base pair sequence.

Its participation in the Human Genome Project helped China to develop the technological capacity to undertake cutting-edge genomic science, and sparked the development of advanced bioinformatics infrastructures and supercomputing facilities needed to support this research. China plans to continue its genomic sequencing efforts through the pig genome project (in collaboration with Danish scientists) and the super-hybrid rice genome sequencing project. It is also supporting a major SNP mapping project and rapidly developing technologies for functional genomics research. The government has reaffirmed its commitment to continuing this drive, announcing an additional $350 million funding for genomics and biotechnology programmes through its priority "863" R&D projects in February 2000.

The development of the technological infrastructure and facilities for world-class genomic science will be invaluable in China's ongoing drive to attract back its most talented scientists from overseas, and benefit from the expertise such individuals have acquired. The

Chinese Academy of Sciences estimate that of over 320,000 scientists who left China to train overseas since 1978, more than two thirds have not returned. There are however signs that major initiatives such as the "300 talents" and "Changjiang Scholars" programmes, which offer enhanced salaries, benefits and research budgets for outstanding scientists are beginning to pay dividends. In 1999, more scientists returned to China than left for overseas positions — the first ever positive flow. Where scientists cannot be tempted back to work full time in China, their skills may be utilized through joint appointments, and grants for short term visits. Increasing levels of funding are being made available to support such mechanisms.

Although these capacity building initiatives have met with tremendous success, a number of key challenges remain. In particular, the lack of investment opportunities for entrepreneurs constitutes a barrier in stimulating the development of a vibrant biotechnology sector.

While China is encouraging research collaborations between its own scientists and those in the developed countries, it is acutely aware of the need to protect its genetic heritage in light of previous malpractice by overseas researchers, which has seen the illegal export of thousands of samples attained from members of the population without proper informed consent. To help counter these concerns, the Human Genetic Resources Administration was established to ensure that collaborative genetic research is based on equal partnerships between local and overseas scientists and that resulting intellectual property rights are shared. China is also initiating educational and public engagement programmes to ensure that scientists, policy-makers and the general public are aware of the ethical implications of genomics research and that these issues are debated widely. Religious groups have been included in these discussions for the first time.

References

1. Anon (2000). China to seek more overseas talent. *Chinese Academy of Sciences Bulletin* (Accessed at http://www.bulletin.ac.cn/ACTION/2000081303.htm Jan 16, 2002)

2. Cyranoski, D (2001). A great leap forward. *Nature* 410: 10–12

3. Nature Editorial (2001). China's hopes and hypes. *Nature* 410: 1

4. Li H (2000): Money and machines fuel China's push in sequencing. *Science* 288: 795–98

5. Normile D (2001). New Incentives Lure Chinese Talent Back Home. *Science* 28: 417–18.

6. Yang H (2001). Paper presented at The Bangkok Multiregional Consultation on Genomics and World Health (23–25 July 2001)

Box 5.6   INDIA — BUILDING BIOTECHNOLOGY CAPACITY AND ENABLING BIOINFORMATICS

In order to further its goal of becoming self reliant in front-line areas and develop the capacity to apply modern biotechnology to local health care priorities and realise the resulting social and economic benefits, the Indian Government established the Department of Biotechnology in 1986. The commitment of the government in facilitating the growth of biotechnology is reflected in the Department's annual budget of approximately US$ 30 million.

The Department supports both capacity strengthening and frontline R&D programmes in areas in which technical capacity exists but for which financial resources are lacking, encouraging collaborative links between academia and industry. The Department is also

Box 5.6 (CONTINUED)

responsible for developing appropriate regulatory standards for biotechnology research in the country. The biotechnology programmes are being implemented through a number of autonomous and statutory institutions and universities which receive grants-in-aid. The success of the Department is demonstrated by its outputs — more than 5000 research publications, 4000 postdoctoral students through 62 MSc Post-Doctoral courses and several technologies transferred to industry have resulted from the programmes it has funded.

The Department has been successful in fostering international and regional collaboration and has developed bilateral biotechnology projects with many countries. It is also co-host to the International Centre for Genetic Engineering and Biotechnology (ICGEB), whose activities are aimed specifically at strengthening the research capability of its members, mostly from developing countries. The ICGEB facility at New Delhi offers advanced training fellowships, collaborative PhD programmes and training workshops and symposia, as well as undertaking an extensive research programme.

Through its programme in Human Genetics and Genome Analysis, the Department of Biotechnology supports research and development activities to utilize the technologies of genomics to problems of importance in India. The programme supports clinical genetics research and genetic services, human genome diversity studies, gene therapy research and a major functional genomics programme at the Centre of Biochemical Technology in New Delhi.

Recently, the government affirmed its support for genomics by initiating a new US$ 4 million per year programme in molecular medicine and genomics through the Indian Council of Medical Research.

Recognising also the importance of information technology for pursuing advanced research in modern biology and biotechnology, the Department of Biotechnology launched a bioinformatics programme in 1986–87. It has built a Biotechnology Information System Network covering practically the whole country, comprising 10 Distributed Information Centres and 46 Sub-Centres around an Apex Centre at the Department. The network has evolved state of the art computational and communication resources and is able to support sophisticated bioinformatics research. It has allowed the development of molecular modelling and other bio computational needs (e.g. software tools for sequence analysis of genes) and also provides the support for the R&D activities in genomics and proteomics. Four long-term training courses at the level of post-MSc Diploma are offered by constituent centres within the network to help address the skill gap in this field.

As a result of the network, a large number of public domain databases in the area of molecular biology and genetic engineering is now available to Indian scientists. Through hosting mirror sites of major databases of international standards, India has thus become a major regional nodal point for various genomic-related databanks and networks.

Reference:

Department of Biotechnology, Ministry of Science and Technology, Government of India. (Website http://dbtindia.nic.in)

Box 5.7   THE ASIA-PACIFIC MOLECULAR BIOLOGY NETWORK: REGIONAL
COLLABORATION TO PROMOTE EXCELLENCE

The Asia-Pacific International Molecular Biology Network (IMBN) was established in
June 1997 by a network of scientists from leading research institutions across Asia and
the Pacific Rim to promote regional cooperation in the development of molecular biology
and biotechnology, and benefit from the considerable potential of these technologies to
improve the economic status of the populations in the region.

The IMBN, which is modelled loosely on the European Molecular Biology Organization
(EMBO), strives to maintain and promote the development of excellence in molecular
biology and biotechnology amongst scientists and institutions in the region and promote
awareness of the importance of this research among policy-makers. In realization of the
multidisciplinary nature of modern biomedical research and the rapid development of
new techniques in the field, the network aims to foster collaborative links between scientists to increase synergies in addressing regional research priorities, maximize the use of
regional facilities and promote skill exchange. The network's activities accommodate the
wide range of existing scientific and technological capabilities across the region, and their
widely divergent historical and cultural backdrops. It has four key objectives, to:

- promote study, research innovation, development and dissemination of knowledge in
  molecular biology, genetic engineering and directly related areas.

- establish facilities and training programs to strengthen expertise and capacity for these
  disciplines.

- coordinate the conduct of research and development activities in laboratories designated by supporting institutions as Asia-Pacific International Molecular Biology
  Laboratories.

- co-operate with industry to identify areas of common interest.

The IMBN strives to work with other international organizations to streamline and coordinate activities targeted towards common goals and minimize duplication of effort. It is
dedicated to promoting excellence in scientific research and its member scientists are
selected on this basis. As of November 2001, 243 world class scientists from its 15 participating economies had been elected as members of the IMBN. An international expert
advisory panel of world leading scientists serves to guide and advise the Governing Body,
which is elected from the members. The IMBN receives funding from supporting institutions across the region, and focuses its activities through designated participating centres
of excellence.

To develop its strategy focus, the IMBN convened a Strategic Vision Commission which
reported in 2000. Concurrently, nine IMBN member countries undertook priority needs
assessments for biotechnology development. These analyses provided a framework to
guide future activities of the IMBN (Table).

The IMBN has initiated a number of programmes to further its aims, including:

- *The Asia-Pacific IMBN Media and Public Education Programme in the Life Sciences*
  — regional courses for young journalists in challenges, opportunities and ethics of
  molecular biology and biotechnology and a public education programme dedicated to
  information, resources and materials to improve educational curricula.

- *A formal partnership with the Asia-Pacific Bioinformatics Network (APBioNet)* to
  implement common programmes in bioinformatics towards the building of core com-
  petencies and resource sharing.

Box 5.7 (CONTINUED)

- *Prospective Industry-Academia Collaborations and Consortia* — promoting industry-academia partnerships aimed at developing areas of common interest and providing suitable fora to facilitate their development.

- *Asia-Pacific IMBN Laboratories* — the IMBN has developed guidelines for the establishment and operation of unit-sized or centralized laboratories in the region.

- *IMBN fellowships and studentships* — for outstanding candidates to undertake short visits to overseas centres of excellence.

References:

1. Ip NY, Shahi G (1999). A molecular biology network for Asia and the Pacific Rim. *Science*, 285:1222–1223.

2. IMBN Web site: http://www.a-imbn.org

PRIORITY NEEDS FOR ASIA-PACIFIC INTERNATIONAL MOLECULAR BIOLOGY NETWORK (IMBN)

Key Success Factor	Issue	Recommendations for IMBN
Infrastructure Development	Varying levels of technological capacity across region. Lack of critical mass of scientists and duplication of resources	Provide guidelines on infrastructure requirements
R&D Culture	Thriving community lacking in smaller or developing economies. Limited entreprenurial atmosphere.	Explore establishment of IMBN supported lab or centre of excellence to facilitate academia-industry relations and scientific exchange
Legislation and IPR (intellectual property right) Protection	Legislation needs to be adaptable and respond to needs of the public. Structures in place but implementation is weak leading to low public awareness and hesitation by industry to invest in R&D.	Education and training initiatives for legislation development and IPR protection. Foster collaboration between scientists policy-makers, legal experts and media
Human Resources	Lack of attractiveness of scientific career paths and dearth of scientific managers in the region.	Cross-training in academia and industry settings Review of career evaluation
Finance and Resource Mobilization	Although public funds are available, evaluation systems are opaque and funding foci change rapidly. Low participation of industry in R&D.	Development of evaluators to aid policy-makers in funding decisions

countries will not to be able to evolve the structure to be able to benefit from the fruits of the postgenomic period, thus widening further the developed-developing country technological and economic gap.

There is a need therefore to initiate a process whereby the pharmaceutical and related industries of developing countries can gain the kind of expertise in biotechnology which is required for application to their own particular health needs. While university-based scientists and those who work in related research institutes can make valuable contributions to these types of research and development programmes, the situation will not be corrected until the pharmaceutical industries of developing countries evolve appropriate capacity in technology and skills. This is a problem of great urgency which requires discussion with the governments and pharmaceutical industries of the developed countries.

One way forward would be the establishment of innovative industrial partnerships between developed and developing countries which could provide both the training and technical expertise required by industry in the developing countries. This would require a great deal of good will on the part of the governments of the developed countries, with the inducement of tax benefits and other incentives to their pharmaceutical industries to encourage partnerships of this kind. These important issues are discussed further in Section 7.

Since some of the developing countries have limited or even non-existent pharmaceutical industries, other approaches to developing partnerships of this type need to be considered. As outlined in Section 2, the plant genome field is starting to pay dividends. For example, in Brazil it is already leading to improvements in the citrus industry from information acquired from the *Xylella* genome project (see Box 5.4). And the potential for a new paradigm in developing insecticides based on genomics is currently gaining momentum. In Pakistan, the National Institute of Biotechnology and Genetic Engineering provides a good example of an institution in which both agriculture *and* health-related research are developing under the same roof and hence frequently utilize common resources. In the light of some of the economic successes arising from plant genomics, and considering the lack of biotechnology expertise in many of the developing countries, together with the limited development of their pharmaceutical industries, there is a strong case for the further exploration of partnerships between agriculture and health-related research in genomics.

The importance of developing dialogues along these lines cannot be over-emphasized. If, as seems likely, genomics does produce major benefits for health, the lack of biotechnological expertise in the pharmaceutical industry in the developing world will lead to a major exacerbation of the inequalities of health care among different countries. WHO has an important role to play in facilitating the types of complex international interactions discussed above.

5.5   FORGING INTERNATIONAL PARTNERSHIPS IN ACADEMIA

While it is clear that many of the potential advances for health that will arise from genomics will need to be developed in industry, there are others which, because they will be of little commercial value, will need to evolve in the university sector and in related research institutions. There is, therefore, an important requirement for forging international partnerships between academic researchers.

The relatively rapid transfer of DNA technology from the developed to the developing countries in the case of the thalassaemias and other inherited disorders of haemoglobin is an excellent example of what can be done by forging strong relationships between universities across the world. These partnerships were established by personal contacts and, perhaps equally importantly, a series of international meetings sponsored by specialist societies and WHO which brought together clinicians and basic scientists with a particular interest in this field. The approach worked well because it was a genuine partnership; the constant exchange of young people for scientific training ensured that the technology was properly transferred and not confined to the laboratories of the developed countries to further their research programmes. There are relatively few incentives for industry to become involved in this type of partnership and it will be very important to further the interaction of universities, governments and charitable research organizations between the developed and developing countries.

There are some constraints to the evolution of this extremely effective pattern of international technology transfer. Naturally, the governments of the developed countries will almost always tend to fund research of the highest priority to their own populations. And while charitable organizations, including the Bill and Melinda Gates Foundation, the John D. and Catherine T. MacArthur and Rockefeller Foundations in the USA, and the Wellcome Trust in the United Kingdom, have done much in this field, without further support on the part of the governments of developed countries it will be difficult for it to expand to the degree that is necessary.

There needs to be a much more global attitude towards medical education and research on part of the universities of the developed countries. With some notable exceptions, the level of training and awareness concerning the problems of the developing countries is very limited in many medical schools. Although increasing numbers of young people are spending elective periods in the developing countries, these programmes need to be enlarged. In addition, there needs to be an increase in expenditure on research in problems relevant to the developing countries by governments and non-governmental organizations in the richer countries.

Another problem which has to be addressed in this context is the fact that commercial interests are increasingly driving the public research agenda in many developed countries. If unchecked, this trend will have a deleterious effect on encouraging scientists in academia from pursuing research directed at improving the health of people living in the developing countries. This problem applies equally to the basic science required for the further understanding of the pathogenesis of the diseases of these countries and to the transitional research required to develop this research for the benefit of their communities.

It is important therefore that WHO takes a lead in increasing international awareness of these complex problems. It could play a major role in encouraging the developed countries to take a more global view of medical education and biomedical research. This could be done by pointing out that, with the potential importance of genomics for improving global health, and the fact that there is likely to be a much more homogenous distribution of illness among different countries in the future, health care and research are international rather than narrow, national activities. Those who administer medical research and education in the developed countries must be made aware of these trends.

5.6 REGIONAL COLLABORATION

As mentioned earlier, several of the developing countries already have well-advanced biotechnology capacities (Section 5.4). And there are encouraging signs that this trend is expanding. For example, in a recent review of the situation in Africa a number of centres of excellence were described and it was reported that several African nations have recently invested in science and technology programmes (Hassan, 2001). In attempting to improve the capacity of the developing countries to enable them to take advantage of the benefits of health care which are likely to result from genomics in the future there is, therefore, increasing scope for regional collaboration. This particularly important aspect of post-genomic health planning should be encouraged further by WHO. The Asia-Pacific International Molecular Biology Network provides an excellent model of a regional approach to capacity building (Box 5.7).

5.7   INFORMATION TECHNOLOGY AND BIOINFORMATICS

The medical developments arising from genome projects will depend on the increasingly sophisticated information technology and bioinformatics required to analyse and interpret the vast amount of data that are being generated. A great deal of this is in the public domain and freely available to those with the facilities and expertise to utilize it. For example, all the information derived from the International Human Genome Sequencing Consortium, the International SNP Map Working Group and many of the international pathogen and model organism genome sequencing consortia is made available immediately to scientists throughout the world. Furthermore, the majority of scientific journals insist on DNA data being deposited in publicly available databases. Increasingly sophisticated algorithm programmes directed at analysing both the genome and the proteome are becoming available, all of which are making it easier and faster to annotate individual genomes. In the commercial sector, Celera allows scientists to view their draft human genome sequence data at no charge, though some constraints are placed on how it is used. Some of the commercial software required for genome analyses is, however, extremely expensive.

Clearly, if the developing countries are not to be left behind in this extraordinary period of development in information technology it is vital that they are able to obtain the computational facilities and technical skills required. Because the field has moved so rapidly, even the developed countries have a major shortage of scientists and technicians in this field. There is also a major shortage of population geneticists with skills in quantitative genetics. Without these personnel however, it will be impossible for countries to develop either strong research bases or their industrial biotechnology bases to a level at which they can be competitive.

This problem is particularly pressing for countries wishing to develop their own pathogen genome projects directed at the communicable diseases which are particularly common in their populations. Hence the field of information technology and bioinformatics presents a particular challenge for a concerted international effort towards training both scientists and technicians with the skills required.

5.8   SUMMARY AND FUTURE POSSIBILITIES

Clearly, genomics has considerable potential for improving the health of the developing countries in the future. As outlined in Section 3, there are many important research programmes arising from pathogen genomics which, if they come to fruition, could be of enormous value in this respect. In particular, the development of new families of vaccines and therapeutic agents, and the ability to genetically manipulate pathogen vectors, could play a major role in controlling communicable disease in the future.

However, there are many unanswered questions. None of these advances will be of any value unless the developing countries can evolve the health care systems on which these new advances can be based. In most cases it is too early to assess the economic consequences of improvements in health care which may stem from genomics as compared with more conventional approaches. Despite the increasing evidence for the globalization of disease, there are still considerable doubts about the will of the governments of developed countries to help to solve health problems which do not appear to be directly germane to their own populations. There is also the concern that, by attempting to apply the advances from genomics to the health of the developing countries at this stage, resources will be used which would be better directed at the provision of basic health care systems. These issues are discussed further in Section 7.

Given the magnitude of these problems, it has been suggested that it may be too early to consider attempting to start to apply the fruits of genomics research to the health of the developing countries. From the examples given in the earlier part of this section it is clear that this is not the case. Provided that a balance is maintained between conventional methods of public health and clinical practice, that each new development is carefully tested with adequate pilot studies, that the best possible use is made of local expertise by networking and the development of developed-developing country partnerships, and that more realistic attitudes on global health on the part of governments and industry of developed countries can be encouraged through the advocacy of international agencies like WHO, a start can and should be made in establishing the foundations on which this new technology can be introduced for the benefit of the developing countries as it becomes available in future years.

6. POTENTIAL RISKS AND HAZARDS OF THE APPLICATIONS OF GENOMICS AND THEIR CONTROL

Contents

6.1 INTRODUCTION

When, in the mid 1970s, it became possible to rearrange and join together pieces of DNA from different species in the test-tube to recreate hybrid molecules, or recombinant DNA, there was considerable public concern, which was also expressed by many scientists, about the potential dangers of this new technology. Moratoria were called, often in haste, and for a while it appeared that the field might not move forward. Doomsday scenarios, in which the catastrophic consequences of experiments involving, for example, the transfer of tumour virus genes into bacteria, became a regular feature in the media. At the Asilomar Conference in 1975 many of these issues were discussed and put into perspective, a process which was continued at further national and international meetings. Experience of this technology over the next 20 years suggested that many of these fears were groundless, although there is still no room for complacency in this complex field. The potential risks and hazards must never be underestimated, and they must be fully addressed, allowing science to progress and society to reap the benefits in safety (Fukuyama, 2002).

The risks of DNA technology and the ways in which they can be contained have been widely publicized. Here we summarize the main principles of the central mechanisms involved, and how they might be applied in countries which are new to this field.

6.2   GENETIC MANIPULATION

Over the last twenty years there has been a gradual evolution of control procedures in countries in which genetic manipulation has become a major research tool. In order to protect both individual scientists and the community from the risks, albeit remote, of the release of harmful pathogens or cancer-producing agents, a series of sensible guidelines and committee structures, backed up where appropriate by legislation, have been established. Where these systems have worked most effectively they have evolved through prolonged debate and interaction between scientists, the public and government, followed by the development of sensible laws and the setting up of regulatory organizations.

In the United Kingdom, for example, the government set up an Advisory Committee on Gene Manipulation and rules and guidelines for recombinant DNA research were established. There was an intensive effort to establish levels of risk assessment and all work of this type is, by law, categorized in this way. Recombinant DNA research must be registered and its safety assessed, and regular visits are made to establishments in which work of this type is being carried out. These institutions must, again by law, have their own biological safety committees, and must monitor carefully and keep full records of all work of this type.

As the field of recombinant DNA technology has expanded, this type of control and legislative process has moved along with it. In the United Kingdom, for example, when somatic-cell gene therapy was likely to become a reality, a government committee on the associated ethical issues was set up, initially to decide whether this field should be pursued at all. Once this was agreed, the Gene Therapy Advisory Committee was established and it was required that the committee should approve all gene therapy protocols before the research is carried out. These decisions have to be agreed by both this national committee and by institutional ethics committees.

Similar regulatory and legal mechanisms have been established in most countries in which work of this type is done. For example, in the USA, the Office of Biotechnology Activities, which is within the Director's Office at the National Institutes of Health (NIH), is a central body responsible for monitoring the application of recombinant DNA technology, genetic testing and other aspects of medical biotechnology. The Office of Biotechnology Activities works through three expert committees: the Recombinant DNA Advisory Committee, the Secretaries Advisory Committee on Genetic Counselling, and the Secretaries Advisory

Committee on Xenotransplantation. Mechanisms of regulation are very similar to those outlined for the United Kingdom, and similar patterns have evolved in many of the developed countries.

This evolutionary process for continually monitoring new developments and for putting in place appropriate control mechanisms is essential in a field which is moving so rapidly. Overall, although it tends to produce new layers of bureaucracy which may slow scientific progress for a while, it is effective. It is vital therefore that the regulatory principles, which have evolved from over 20 years experience, are made available to countries in which recombinant DNA technology is either in the early days of its development or has not yet been established. Also, if developed-developing country collaborations are to become an important catalyst in helping the latter countries to evolve this technology, the establishment of sound regulatory principles must be achieved as soon as possible in these countries. The important advisory role for a central body like WHO in helping to establish guidelines of this type is self-evident.

6.3   RISKS IN NON-HUMAN GENOMICS
6.3.1   *Animals and insects*

A great deal of work is being carried out using recombinant DNA technology to alter the genome of a wide variety of animals and insects to try to create animal models of disease, to produce diagnostic and therapeutic agents, or to disable disease-carrying vectors. As discussed in Section 3, the creation of animals with specific genetic disorders also facilitates the analysis of normal and abnormal gene function and, by outbreeding, provides a valuable approach to the further identification of genes which may modify human genetic diseases.

Genetically modified (GM) animals are being engineered to produce in their milk or tissues therapeutic agents of benefit to humans, including blood clotting factors, antibodies, human albumin and a variety of hormones. Strains of animals particularly prone to develop diseases like cancer are being generated for testing anticancer agents or screening for environmental carcinogens. In agriculture, GM animals are being developed primarily to generate disease-resistant forms or to produce desirable alterations to growth rates or feed conversion efficiency. GM insects that spread human pathogens are being modified such that they are incapable of transmitting disease. The aim is to replace a wild population with strains that could reduce or eliminate disease transmission.

This new area of research poses a number of potential hazards, including the evolution of new or increased allergic reactions in humans to animals used as a food source, toxic effects on the environment from the production of new biologically active proteins, adverse effects to other animals from changes in behaviour; alterations in the ability of an animal to act as a human disease reservoir; and the effect on the ecosystem of releasing genetically modified animals or insects into the environment. There are also concerns about the remote possibility of inserting foreign genes into the human genome from animal sources derived through these routes.

While work in the broad area of genetic modification undoubtedly has important potential for medical research and the improvement of human health, like all forms of recombinant DNA technology, it requires careful monitoring and control. In many countries regulatory bodies are taking on this role. In the United Kingdom for example, the Advisory Committee on Genetic Modification has legal powers to regulate, licence and monitor all experiments involving genetic modification. No experiments of this type can be carried out without appropriate licensing and similar legislation is in place for monitoring experiments on invertebrates. The European Community directive on the deliberate release of genetically modified organisms into the environment secures protection of human health and the environment. Recently, a Xenotransplantation Interim Regulatory Authority has been developed in the United Kingdom for the purpose of regulating experiments directed at modifying animals so that their organs might be used for replacing those of diseased organs in humans, with all the adherent risks involved. Equally stringent legislation has been developed in the USA and many European countries to ensure the welfare of animals modified in this way. However, a great deal of research is required before it is clear how much suffering genetic modification will cause to animals and this field requires constant monitoring.

It seems very likely that research of this kind will expand rapidly in the next few years. It raises extremely important safety issues and it is vital that effective regulatory systems and education programmes are available to countries in which this work is not yet developed, but where it is proposed to pursue it in the future.

6.3.2   Plants

The regulation of the safety of GM foods is of great importance for global health. The problems of using conventional toxicology approaches for the evaluation of novel foods was recognized more than 10 years ago and a variety of new approaches have been developed by WHO, Organisation for Economic Cooperation and Development (OECD), and the Food and Agriculture Organization (FAO). The recommendations of these bodies are based largely on the principle of substantial equivalence, which involves the use of a comparative approach to reveal intended and unintended differences between GM food and its untreated counterpart using a substantial body of phenotypic data. It should be emphasized that substantial equivalence is not a safety evaluation and is not intended to identify hazards but rather to reveal differences with respect to an established benchmark which will then become the basis for a further detailed safety evaluation (Gasson and Burke, 2001).

The spectrum of safety issues concerning GM food is extremely wide: the use of microbial and fungal cells as factories for the production of processing enzymes and additives; the potential effects of introducing foreign DNA into plants including the use of bacterial antibiotic resistance genes as selection markers; the risk that transgenic DNA is transferred to the host and might lead to genetic alteration of the host; and the possibility that microorganisms that inhabit the gastrointestinal tract or soil might acquire transgenic DNA. Although many safeguards have been integrated into programmes which might be associated with problems of this kind there are other difficulties in monitoring the effects of GM foods, particularly assessing their effects within human populations. The sources of food are so diverse that increased risks, allergy for example, may be very difficult to relate to any particular modified food.

Although a great deal more research directed at the safety and methods of regulating GM food is required these problems should be put into perspective. A recent authoritative review on this field pointed out that "it is relevant to emphasize that this safety evaluation is far more thorough than that which is applied to new food materials produced by conventional plant breeding that have been safely introduced into the food chain over decades" (Gasson and Burke, 2001).

6.4 CHANGING THE GENETIC CONSTITUTION OF INDIVIDUALS OR POPULATIONS

There has been considerable discussion about the potential dysgenic effects of recombinant DNA technology, particularly as they relate to the control and treatment of genetic disease. These concerns are based on the notion that in our attempts to help families or individuals with a genetic disease we may increase the number of deleterious genes in the human gene pool.

The approaches to the control or treatment of genetic disease were outlined in Section 3. In short, they include preconceptual counselling, prenatal or preimplantation diagnosis, somatic-cell gene therapy, and germ-line gene therapy.

These issues are extremely complex and can only be discussed in outline here. Preventing parents who are carrying the same genetic defect from reproducing, and hence having affected children, will tend to interfere with the normal evolutionary mechanism for reducing the frequency of deleterious genes within a population. In offering similarly affected parents the possibility of prenatal diagnosis and termination of pregnancies of affected babies, and thus encouraging them to have children, more carriers will be produced. On the other hand, in the past, families who had children with severe genetic diseases often tended to increase their size as a compensatory mechanism; since the instigation of prenatal diagnosis for thalassaemia in Mediterranean populations, family sizes have fallen to more or less match the population norm. Of course, pre-implantation diagnosis, with exclusion of doubly affected or carrier embryos, would solve some of these problems.

Whichever approach is taken, however, it will take many generations to produce any significant change in the frequency of genetic diseases in the population by these interventions, and most geneticists do not feel that current technology offers a serious risk to the human gene pool (Neel, 2000). On the other hand, if it becomes more widespread it is something that will have to be monitored carefully.

Unlike somatic-cell gene therapy, the successful development of germ-line gene therapy might have a more immediate effect on the human gene pool. Somatic-cell gene therapy aimed at serious genetic disease can, with careful regulation, obtain reasonable risk-benefit ratios. However, it has been argued that germ-line gene therapy, because its effects will be passed on to successive generations, cannot satisfy the necessary risk-benefit ratios to be allowed to go forward.

It is important to distinguish whether germ-line therapy is now sufficiently safe to be permitted from whether it could become so in the future. At present, it is not possible to remove and replace a gene at the correct place on the chromosome. Instead, it must be delivered on a crude, imprecise vector that may generate unintended genetic effects with unknown risks (see Section 3.9). If gene therapy is aimed at multifactorial diseases, as opposed to single- gene disorders, both the likelihood of technical error as well as the difficulty of predicting how genes or their products interact with each other increases exponentially. Moreover, some of the research necessary to limit these risks may require human experimentation that would be difficult to perform ethically.

For these and other reasons there is widespread consensus that germ-line gene therapy, because its potential harmful consequences would be passed on to future generations, should not be permitted at the present time, even in the case of serious genetic disease. The risk-benefit ratio of germ-line interventions would be even less favourable in the case of less serious genetic disease or in the case of genetic enhancement.

In somatic-cell gene therapy, on the other hand, these risks are limited to the individual on whom the therapy is performed, which both limits their potential effects and often allows for the individual to decide whether to consent to undertake the risks. However, it is possible that at some point in the future gene therapy may have progressed to the point at which germ-line gene therapy, particularly for serious genetic disease, promises a sufficiently favourable risk-benefit ratio to warrant its use. When it is clearly desirable to prevent serious disease in a particular individual, it could likewise be desirable to prevent that disease in future generations as well. This implies that permanent bans on germ-line gene therapy may not be justified.

6.5 GENETIC DATABASES

The planned development of large-scale genetic databases offers a series of hazards and ethical issues which have not been previously encountered. Here the general nature of these databases and some of the potential hazards are briefly outlined. The ethical issues involved are discussed briefly in Section 8.

The concept of genetic databases is not new. For the last 30 years it has been common practice to establish registers of patients with genetic diseases, aimed at providing genetic services to families with these conditions. For example, the Register for the Ascertainment and Prevention of Inherited Disease in Edinburgh, Scotland offered members of families with genetic disease active counselling as soon as they reached adulthood. Similarly, a register centred at the University of Utah, UT, USA was based on the family register of the Mormon Church to identify individuals with autosomal dominant hypercholesterolemia, a condition with a high risk of early myocardial infarction and death. Recently, a national database for families with thalassaemia has been established in the United Kingdom (Modell et al., 2001). Clearly these genetic registers greatly benefit individuals, families and societies.

The new generation of genetic databases are quite different, both in size, scope, and format. In many cases they involve extremely large populations (Box 6.1). For example, the Icelandic Health Sector Database aims to link health records with genealogical information and information about genotype. The objective is to facilitate research on the genetic factors in common diseases. DNA samples will be collected with informed consent, whereas entry into the health records database is by presumed consent. This project involves a single commercial company which will receive any potential profits from discoveries that come from the database, some of which will be fed back into health provision for Icelanders. Another example is the proposed United Kingdom Population Biomedical Collection which will be based on samples and data from 500,000 adults aged between 45 and 60 years and, again, its aim is to help to establish the genetic and environmental factors involved in common diseases such as cancer and cardiovascular disease. Informed consent of volunteers will be sought and no single company will be granted exclusive access; samples will be held in public ownership. In both cases data will be stored in a form that will not allow researchers to identify individuals.

There is still considerable controversy about the desirability of establishing databases of this type and there are many ambiguities regarding access and control. Concerns are focused on the potential harm to individuals, groups and communities. Concerns about individual risks revolve around those arising from access to genetic information, both by individuals themselves and by third parties. The latter might include health insurance companies, government bodies, or the legal profession and police. Hence a great deal of attention is being paid to the questions of confidentiality and access to these databases. Although much effort is being put into protecting individuals there are still possibilities for the misuse of the databases.

It has also been suggested that genetic research based on these collections may have the effect of stigmatizing entire countries or particular groups of individuals, and there are concerns about commercial exploitation without adequate compensation. Also, because scientific research depends on freedom of access to samples and information, the commercial ownership of these databases may have a deleterious effect on genetic research. As well as these concerns, there are a variety of economic and

Box 6.1   POPULATION GENETIC DATABASES: ICELAND, ESTONIA AND TONGA

The Icelandic Health Sector Database

Several factors combine to make Iceland a particularly attractive environment in which to study the genetics and epidemiology of complex human disease. The lack of immigration and a number of marked population bottlenecks over the last 1100 years mean that the present population of 285 000 individuals has a particularly high degree of genetic homogeneity. Iceland has a universal and well-funded national health care system and well-maintained medical records stretching back approximately a century. Furthermore, levels of education are high and the public is for the most part highly supportive of scientific research.

The Centralized Health Sector Database Act was presented to Althingi (the Icelandic Parliament) in March 1998, and adopted into law in a revised form in December 1998. The Act is for the establishment of a research resource containing selected health data from the medical records of the Icelandic population, stored in a coded (anonymized) format. It does not provide for the collection of genetic data or biological samples. Although approved by Parliament over three years ago, the resource has yet to become operational.

The submission of data from individual medical records will be by presumed consent, however an opt-out mechanism has been established to enable individuals to withhold their medical data if they so chose. By December, 2001 approximately 20 000 Icelandic citizens had chosen to exercise this right. All data will undergo a two-stage encryption process to ensure that it is non-identifiable to research users. This process will be under the strict control of the Icelandic Data Protection Commission, and the operation of the resource will be overseen by the National Bioethics Committee.

The Act decreed that an exclusive 12-year license be granted to a private company to establish and utilize the data for the purposes of genetic association studies, diagnostic and drug development and improving health care management. In January 2000, the Ministry of Health announced that an Iceland-based biotechnology company, deCODE Genetics, was to receive this operating licence. In 1998, deCODE had entered into partnership with the Swiss pharmaceutical company, Hoffmann LaRoche, who contributed US$ 200 million for the right to develop drugs for 12 common diseases, based on genes mapped by deCODE as the result of cohort studies in Iceland. The sale of US$ 2 million of deCODE shares to Icelanders in 1998 further enhanced Iceland's stake in the company.

In establishing the resource, deCODE will negotiate terms with individual health care institutions for collating the encrypted data from medical records. Through these arrangements, deCODE is contributing to the development of medical informatics infrastructures at the proposed data resource centres for the benefit of national health care planning and management. Future plans for the resource include linking the medical record data in the Health Sector Database to the extensive genealogical data which Iceland possesses and to genetic data collected from research participants through full voluntary informed consent.

It must be acknowledged that concerns have been raised over the proposed resource by a number of commentators from academic and clinical medicine both in Iceland and internationally. Particular concerns include the appropriateness of presumed consent, the effects that the opt-out procedure will have on representativity, the lack of public debate in the initial drafting of the Database Act and the extent to which Icelandic academics will be able to access the data. Despite these concerns, it seems clear that the Icelandic public are supportive of the initiative as shown by the huge majority support in public opinion polls.

Box 6.1 (CONTINUED)

A wide ranging consultative and public debate process has been underway since the initiative was announced in 1998. Agreement was finally reached in late 2001between the official representatives of the medical profession, government and DeCode to proceed together for 12 years.

The Estonian Genome Project

The idea of a population genetic database in Estonia was first proposed in 1999 by the Estonian Genome Foundation, a consortium of national scientists. The projected goal of the resource is to create a database collating genotype and phenotype data for at least three quarters of the 1.4 million people of the country. The project will involve the collection of blood samples from patients for SNP (single nucleotide polymorphisms) analysis, together with clinical histories and genealogical information.

The estimated cost of establishing the proposed resource will be between US$ 100 and US$ 150 million over a five year period. Although the Estonian government has pledged substantial funds, it is planned that the majority of these costs will be met through private investment, from Estonian and international sources.

The samples and data will be owned and managed by the Estonian Genome Project Foundation (EGPF), a not-for-profit organization, established by the Estonian Genome Foundation and Ministry of Health. The EGPF has established a for-profit subsidiary (EGeen) to serve as an investment vehicle. EGeen will seek strategic alliances and negotiate non-exclusive license agreements with pharmaceutical and biotechnology companies to access the encrypted data for research purposes. Estonian academics will be able to access the data for free or for a minimal handling fee.

As a crucial step in planning the resource, a legal and ethical framework for its operation was developed as detailed in the Human Genes Research Act, which was passed by the Estonian parliament in December 2000. The Act includes the following provisions:

- All samples must be stored in Estonia.
- Participation in the project is by voluntary informed consent.
- Participants may remove data at any time.
- All information in the database will be encrypted via a 16-digit code system.
- The information may not be used for discriminatory purposes.
- An ethics committee will be established to oversee the operation of the resource.

A US$ 5 million pilot project on cancer genetics was to begin in autumn 2001. This project aims to collect samples and clinical information from 10 000 patients and serve as a forerunner to the creation of the resource.

The Population Database of Tonga

In November 2000, it was announced that the Tongan Ministry of Health had entered into discussions with an Australian biotechnology company, Autogen to establish a genetic database resource for the 108,000 population of the island with the aim of identifying genes involved in common diseases.

In the deal, Autogen is to establish a research facility in the Tongan capital, Nuku'Alofa and provide annual research funding to the health ministry. The DNA samples collected

Box 6.1 (CONTINUED)

will remain the property of Tonga and be housed locally, but Autogen will have exclusive access rights for commercial useage of the data.

Autogen has pledged that full voluntary informed consent will be obtained from individuals and that all information will undergo an encryption process. Furthermore, any therapeutic products that result will be made freely available to the Tongan people and 1–3% of profits from the research fed back to Tonga as recommended in the HUGO (Human Genome Organization) Statement on Benefit Sharing. The data will be freely available to the Tongan people to use in health management and public health policy-making. An Ethics Committee will be established to oversee the project. As of early 2002 there is no confirmation of the agreement between Autogen and Tonga.

The Tongan case has raised several concerned responses. For example, the Tongan Human Rights and Democracy Movement spoke out in condemnation of the agreement. In March 2001, the Pacific Council of Churches released a consensus statement asserting the rights of the peoples of the Pacific, as "guardians of their heritage" to manage their own biological resources and protect them from exploitation. It recommends that governments must facilitate full public consultation when any genetic research project is proposed, make all relevant information available, engage independent experts and prepare regional legislation to safeguard biopiracy and related issues.

References

1. Position paper presented by Dr Sigurdur Gudmundsson at the ACHR Consultation on Genomics and Health (Geneva, 27 June 2001)

2. Rose H. (2001), The commodification of bioinformation: The Icelandic Health Sector Database. London, The Wellcome Trust.

3. Icelandic Ministry of Health and Social Security, http://brunnur.stjr.is/interpro/htr/htr.nsf/pages/forsid-ensk

4. DeCODE Genetics website: www.decode.com

5. Estonian Genome Foundation, http://www.genome.ee

6. Autogen website: http://www.autogenlimited.com.au

7. Official Statements: Genetic research in Tonga. Bulletin of Medical Ethics, 166, 8–10.

8. Burton B (2002). Proposed genetic database on Tongans opposed. *British Medical Journal*, 324:443.

ethical issues posed by this new trend in genetic science (see Sections 7 and 8; Chadwick and Berg, 2001).

Another major issue about the establishment of large-scale databases is that some developing countries are establishing collections of this type, often at the behest of companies from the developed world. Because of the lack of appropriate regulatory and ethical bodies in some of these developing countries these problems become much more serious and the dangers of inequitable commercial exploitation are even more acute.

Many countries now have DNA databases containing DNA from convicted criminals. The use of DNA testing for forensic purposes also raises a number of important issues which have yet to be settled. Just some of these are: should DNA testing be compulsory for those being investigated for criminal activities?; How long should samples be stored in databases?; Should members of the public be asked to donate DNA for "elimination" purposes? (Reilly, 2001). Currently a United States National Commission is studying these complex issues.

Although these new approaches to medical research and forensic practice, arising directly from genomics, have great potential for improving our understanding of the pathogenesis of common disease and for decreasing crime rates, they raise a number of issues that require further attention. Due to the fact they are very recent developments it is still too early to put them into perspective but it is clearly an area of research and development in health care and public policy which must be very carefully monitored by the international health community. It is not certain whether individuals who donate DNA samples for these databases are fully aware of the potential risks involved, and it is even less clear whether some of the arrangements that have been made with the private sector, which is becoming increasingly involved in these enterprises, are adequately controlled. It is also not apparent how information, particularly unexpected findings, will be handled in these large population studies and how these DNA samples will be used above and beyond the stated aims of those who are establishing the databases.

6.6   BIOLOGICAL WARFARE AND OTHER POLITICAL MISUSES

Just as in any scientific revolution, and as well evidenced by physics at the beginning of the 20th century, the potential for political misuse is ever present. The recombinant DNA era undoubtedly offers wide opportunities for the enhancement of the technology of germ warfare, mass destruction of crops, and release of GM organisms or animals into the community for destructive purposes. Similarly, the misuse of genetics leading to a resurgence of eugenics for political gains, discussed in Section 8, remains a matter for concern.

Information which is being derived from the pathogen genome projects is particularly open to abuse. Some of the central objectives of this work, notably the identification of virulence genes and the mechanisms whereby pathogens are able to evade host defence mechanisms, and the increasing ease with which it is possible to manipulate the genomes of bacteria and viruses, while having enormous potential for the betterment of health, provides a broad range of ammunition for those who would misuse this technology. Vulnerability to biological agents is at least in part due to current inability to detect the presence of the agents in time for appropriate isolation or, when available, early treatment for affected individuals. It is hoped that rapid detection methods based on molecular technologies such as PCR will go some way to solving this problem. Similarly, the use of genomics is likely to facilitate the development of vaccines and the development of new therapeutic agents.

The potential misuse of genomics and biotechnology goes beyond pathogen genomics. Plant genomics, which again offers enormous potential for improving our well-being, is equally open to abuse. Recent advances in the cell biology of receptors and bioregulators and the functions of the immune system also open new pathways for biological warfare. The development of technologies to carry out what is sometimes called "directed molecular evolution," in which genes are cut into smaller pieces and then shuffled to produce progeny with completely new properties, may be able to accelerate more classical combinatorial techniques more than 20 fold. While the potential use of this technique to enhance the properties of proteins could provide significant benefits for medical research, it could have serious implications for biowarfare. These and many other possibilities for the misuse of genomics in this way are discussed in detail by Fraser and Dando (2001).

The misuse of biology for any purpose is prohibited by the 1975 Biological and Toxin Weapons Convention (BTWC). The first Article of the Convention prohibits the development, production, stock piling, acquisition or retention of microbial or other biological agents, or toxins of types or in quantities that have no justification for prophylactic, protective or other peaceful purposes. These prohibitions are now accepted by over 140 States Party to the Convention. Unfortunately, however, the States Party did not agree to effective verification procedures; these important issues were debated at the 5th Review Conference of the BTWC at the end of 2001. WHO will also be publishing the second edition of *Health aspects of biological and chemical weapons* at about the same time.

It is vital that the urgency of the bioweapons issue is appreciated and that a uniform mechanism for the verification of the control of pathogens and their manipulation is agreed. It is the scale of this problem which makes regulation and monitoring so difficult. For example, it has been estimated recently that up to 300 universities and several dozen more state or federal government laboratories in the USA currently handle material classified as "select agents" by the federal Centres for Disease Control and Prevention (Malakoff and Enserink, 2001). While this may be an extreme case, there is no doubt that many countries have a similar diversity of institutions that hold pathogens or potential pathogens of one kind or another.

From a practical viewpoint, it would not be possible to bring advances in genomics to a halt because of these risks of political misuse, nor would it be justified to do so given the very great potential for human health and well-being from future advances in this field. However, it is vital that a major international effort is made without delay to provide guidelines for the more effective containment of pathogens and for the regulation of human and pathogen genomics with a potential for such misuse.

Equally importantly, it is essential that the biomedical research community takes a much more serious attitude to the risks of biological warfare. What are the risk-benefit ratios of some of its current genetic engineering procedures? Is it doing all it can to ensure that its work is adequately contained and monitored? Are some of the questions being addressed of sufficient biological importance to be worth the risks involved? If it does not make a major effort to regulate its own activities, it may find that government and international agencies have to be more proactive. If this happens, the resulting bureaucratic mechanisms may well hamper the development of a field which has much to offer for the benefit of global health.

6.7   STEM CELL GENE THERAPY

Approaches to research in stem cell gene therapy, and its potential benefit for the management of a number of intractable diseases, were outlined in Section 3.10. Much of the work in this field is directed at a better understanding of the properties of human embryonic stem cells and how they might be cultured and directed to differentiate into different tissues that could be used for therapeutic grafting. Work of this kind requires a source of human embryos and currently much of it is carried out using embryos that are left over after in vitro fertilization procedures. Based on both their ethical and social considerations the laws regarding embryo research differ widely from country to country (Box 6.2).

If it is found possible to direct the differentiation of human embryonic stem cells into different tissues in culture, and if this work develops

---

Box 6.2   EXAMPLES OF CURRENT LEGISLATION FOR RESEARCH ON EMBRYOS AND CLONING

Embryo Research

UNITED KINGDOM

Research permitted on embryos up to 14 days of development for research on infertility, contraception, birth defects and stem cell therapy (therapeutic cloning). Reproductive cloning is banned.

FRANCE

Prohibits research on embryos requiring their destruction.

GERMANY

Prohibits research on embryos requiring their destruction.

AUSTRALIA

Varies between States. Banned in Victoria, but permitted in New South Wales and Queensland if carried out under regulations of the Australian Medical Research Council. However, in Victoria work on human embryos imported from other countries is permitted.

USA

Complex situation. The US Congress has banned federal funding for human embryo research. However, the ban does not cover research on human embryonic stem cells that have been obtained using private funds, provided that the National Institutes of Health guidelines for how these cells were derived are followed and that the cell lines were derived before August 2001. These issues will be discussed again in 2002.

Cloning: Therapeutic and Reproductive

Many countries have banned reproductive cloning. Some states in the USA and Australia have banned cloning without making the distinction between reproductive and therapeutic cloning. The Council of Europe's Convention on Human Rights and Biomedicine, and UNESCO's Universal Declaration on the Human Genome and Human Rights have banned only reproductive cloning.

(Source. Robertson, A.J. (2001))

---

to the stage at which it has genuine therapeutic possibilities, major new issues will arise which will require wide debate and possible legislation for their control. For example, the number of "spare" embryos derived from in vitro fertilization may not be sufficient to meet the needs of stem cell therapy. Also, as discussed in Section 3, stem cell banks of this kind would raise the serious problem of providing tissue which was not compatible with that of potential recipients. Hence, a great deal of work is now being directed at the possibility of activating individual adult nuclei by inserting them into anucleated eggs. If research along these lines continues, and if it were successful, the availability of sufficient numbers of eggs will undoubtedly become a major problem. Would it be either ethically or practically possible, by appropriate hormone treatment, to ask women to act as donors for eggs for this purpose? Should other sources be used, cadavers or aborted fetuses for example? Or would it be necessary to try to obtain eggs from animal sources for this purpose? Some of the ethical issues which arise from this new field of research are outlined in Section 8. Several countries are presently passing laws to control various aspects of this work (see Box 6.2).

Research in this field is moving so rapidly that it has been very difficult to develop an adequate ethical debate, let alone sensible legislation, to even start to deal with some of the important issues it raises. Clearly this is an area of research which WHO must consider very carefully in the immediate future and be in the position to offer Member States advice on the extremely complex ethical and legal problems involved.

6.8   SUMMARY

Like any new field of biological science genomics is associated with a broad range of potential risks, at least some of which require careful attention to regulation on the part of governments, research institutes, universities, and industry. There is an increasingly strong case for the development of some uniformity of approach to regulatory programmes across the countries of the world. This will require strong leadership by WHO and related international health agencies.

The potential misuse of genomics for the purposes of biowarfare is of particular importance in this respect and an international agreement on guidelines for the most effective ways of monitoring the storage and manipulation of pathogens, and for assessing the effectiveness of these mechanisms, is urgently required. Equally importantly, the biomedical research community must take a much more proactive role in controlling the hazards associated with the misuse of genomics for biowarfare.

While genomics research offers considerable possibilities for the improvement of human health, because it is a new and rapidly evolving field the full extent of its possible hazards are not yet fully appreciated. While much has been learnt about appropriate mechanisms for regulating research and development in this field, it is very important that these lessons are transmitted to countries in which work of this type is just developing. There are major opportunities for developed-developing country collaboration towards achieving this end and to achieving at least some degree of uniformity in the regulation of all aspects of genetic manipulation.

7. Justice and Resource Allocation: Implications for the Post-Genomic Era

Contents

7.1 INTRODUCTION

Throughout the consultations which preceded this Report fears were voiced that the potential benefits that may arise from the genomic revolution, because of the advanced technology and costs which may be required to bring them to fruition, will further exacerbate the inequities of health care between the developing and developed countries. Clearly, this is an absolutely central issue in any discussion on the likely effects of research in genomics on global health in the future.

In Section 5 the importance for the developing countries of evolving the biotechnology and bioinformatic capacity to enable them to take advantage of developments arising from genomics, particularly in the field of communicable disease, was stressed. Also discussed were some of the approaches which might be taken to achieve this end and the difficulties that might be encountered. Here, after summarizing the present inequities in health status and disease burden between the developed and developing countries, some of the major issues which might prevent the developing countries from benefiting from the improvements in health care that may result from genomics, together with potential solutions, are discussed in more detail. Some of the issues raised in this section, particularly relating to the economics of research and development and provision of health care, are the subject of a recent report from the Commission on Macroeconomics and Health (2001).

7.2   CURRENT INEQUITIES IN THE PROVISION OF HEALTH CARE

7.2.1   *Inequities in health status and disease burden*

As we enter the new millennium, fundamental social and economic disparities between the developed and developing countries continue to exist, and in some cases grow even wider. While life expectancies in the developed countries are in the 75–80 year range, in the least developed countries they are only around 40–50 years (UNDP 2001). Low- and middle-income countries account for 85% of the world's population, but 92% of the global disease burden (WHO 1999). Furthermore, this gap is seen to be growing wider as, for example, in the trend of increasing child malnutrition rates in African countries as compared to a decreasing trend in the rest of the world through the 1980s and up until the mid 1990s (WHO Programme of Nutrition, 1997). The majority of deaths among children less than five years old in all developing countries continue to be preventable, with malnutrition as an underlying cause.

Within countries, the poor and marginalized groups bear disproportionately heavier burdens of disease, ill-health and mortalities. Aggregating across 47 countries, the probability of dying between birth and five years of age was estimated to be 4.3–4.8 times higher for poverty groups compared to non-poverty groups (WHO, 1999).

Across much of the developing world communicable diseases constitute the greatest component of the total disease burden, and the control of infectious diseases remains the key challenge for health services. For most African countries for example, infectious diseases are the overwhelming health care priority, with HIV/AIDS, malaria and tuberculosis constituting the greatest health burden. However, in many other developing countries, the pattern of disease is shifting increasingly towards multifactorial "lifestyle" diseases, such as cancer, heart disease and diabetes. Within the developing world, countries find themselves at different stages along this transition. China, Malaysia, and Thailand, for example, are in a transitional state and suffer a double burden from both communicable diseases and lifestyle diseases. Across much of southeast Asia, infectious diseases remain the major health problems, but lifestyle diseases are becoming increasingly prominent.

While the rate of occurrence for communicable diseases and maternal, perinatal and nutritional disorders is 13 times higher in low- and middle- income countries than in high-income countries, the rate of disease burden for non-communicable diseases, taken as a whole, is similar for both (WHO, 1999). Genetic diseases, particularly the thalassemias and glucose-6-phosphate deficiency (G6PD), also represent a significant and growing health problem in developing countries (see Sections 3 and 5).

Whether it is communicable or non-communicable disease, however, the prevalence is usually higher among the lower social classes and poverty groups, in both developed and developing countries. The risk of diabetes and impaired glucose tolerance, for example, has been found to be highest among populations in developing countries and the disadvantaged communities in the developed countries (see Section 5), while the rates for cardiovascular disease are higher among the lower social classes when compared to the upper social classes in developed countries. In addition, HIV/AIDS, although common to both the developed and the developing countries, is considered to have the greatest urgency in the least developed countries and among the poorest and most marginalized groups.

These inequities of health status and disease burden reflect the fact that in the world's least developed countries basic health care infrastructure is lacking. Safe water supply and the provision of primary health care through a network of health centres, which would do much towards improving their health status, do not exist. Even when vaccines or drugs are available many of these countries lack the health care delivery infrastructure necessary for their distribution among their communities.

In the light of these problems, it is not surprising that a recurring concern that emerged from the consultations that preceded this Report was the large-scale channelling of global resources into genomics research at a time when such glaring omissions in primary health services and problems of access to health care remain so widespread.

7.2.2 Issues of development and poverty alleviation

Another key message from the consultations leading up to this Report was that questions of access and equity in genomics cannot be addressed in isolation from broader economic problems, and that the application of genomics in developing countries will achieve little unless there are parallel efforts aimed at development, with attendant improvements in education, the status of women, awareness of the importance of advances in the provision of health care on the part of the population, and many related issues. In short, it was argued that it is crucial that, in countries where it is introduced, genomics research forms part of a wider, integrated strategy to address the determinants of ill health.

A broad and integrated economic development strategy is exemplified by the Millenium Africa Recovery Plan. Known also as the New African

Initiative, it was spearheaded by the Presidents of Algeria, Nigeria and South Africa. It was designed to break the cycle of poverty and underdevelopment, and requires international support for debt cancellation, opening of markets for African goods, and increased investment, while pledging the practice of good governance in order to achieve a climate of peace and stability. The development of health care systems and health research should be more achievable and sustainable within such a strategy, and it would then be possible for the African peoples to benefit from genomics research and its applications.

Clearly, research in genomics and its application has to be considered in the context of an entire health system, of which health research is only one, albeit critical, component. To implement genomics successfully, countries must also develop complementary expertise in a variety of disciplines including epidemiology, health informatics, health finance, health management and health policy. Each of these facets will be required in the assessment of whether it is appropriate to implement a new technology or intervention in the context of individual national health systems. In Thailand, for example, a strategic recommendation has been made to invest 3% of the national health budget in an independently-managed health research programme, which will consider genomics in the context of national health priorities.

Another common problem is that the outcomes of research are not always effectively translated into political action. It was suggested during the Bangkok, Thailand multi-regional consultation (Annex B2.3) that a missing and essential link between knowledge generated from research and political action is lack of societal engagement. Once this has been achieved, political action will follow. Societal engagement activities might include media campaigns, public education, national surveys and regional meetings, and even culminate in social movements. This model has been coined "the triangle that moves the mountain," the three points of the triangle being research knowledge, societal engagement, and political action (Wasi, 2001). It emphasizes the importance of engaging civil society in bridging the gap between health research and its application to improving health and health care access.

A similar concept was enunciated at the Brasilia, Brazil consultation (Annex B2.2), where the hope was expressed that progress in genomics should eventually lead to better health outcomes and improved health care. In order for this to be achieved, the democratization of knowledge needs to take place, whereby communities engage in interactive dialogue with researchers and policy-makers and participate in decision-making about genomics research and its applications. The process of engagement will enable various stakeholders and communities collectively to determine and guide the direction of genomics research and its applications for the public good.

7.3 RESEARCH PRIORITIES AND ACCESS TO THE BENEFITS OF RESEARCH

7.3.1 *The gap between developed and developing countries in health research*

The "10/90 gap" has been used to refer to the wide disparity in global spending on health research between developed and developing countries (Global Forum for Health Research, 2000). There are fears that this gap will be exacerbated further by the genomics revolution. Genomics research, in which entire genomes are sequenced and analysed to elucidate knowledge of gene structure and function, involves the large-scale creation and utilisation of databases through a high level of automation, and therefore requires high capital investment. As such, it has been carried out primarily in developed countries, in both public and private sectors. There have been some notable exceptions, Brazil, China and India, for example (see Boxes 5.4, 5.5. and 5.6). Even so, the investments of these governments are very small when compared to those of the developed countries.

In the developed countries, although much of genomics research was initially undertaken in the public sector, a recent survey reports that private-company spending on genomics has overtaken and is now substantially higher than government and not-for-profit spending (Box 7.1).

The concentration of research funding in the developed countries as well as in the private sector has implications for the determination of research priorities and for access to the products of research. Research priorities in the private sector are driven by market considerations and the profit motive. The private sector does not invest in research aimed at diagnostics or therapeutics for diseases that are predominant in developing countries because the populations that are afflicted and most likely to need them do not have purchasing power. In order to ensure high returns on their investments, companies tend to focus their research and development efforts on products aimed at diseases and health problems that are most prevalent among the populations of the developed countries. In 1997, for example, it was estimated that low- and medium-income coun-

Box 7.1   THE WORLD SURVEY OF FUNDING FOR GENOMICS RESEARCH

In May 2000, a global survey of genomics funding was initiated by the Stanford-in-Washington Programme, supported by a grant from the Burroughs Wellcome Fund. The survey authors drew on empirical data, which are summarized below. Their main conclusion is that "without explicit attention at the international level, the initial technological fruits of genomics are likely to consist primarily of therapeutic and diagnostic applications for conditions affecting large populations in rich countries."

The study comprised a cross-sectional analysis of genomics funding in both public and private sector institutions, together with an analysis of the underlying trends in financial input and scientific outputs of genomics, as revealed by publicly available data on private R&D funding, patent ownership and on the market values of publicly traded firms. The results of the study were reported to the International Conference on Health Research for Development in Bangkok, Thailand in October 2000, and are freely available on the project web site.

The data should be interpreted in light of several caveats — the response rates to the surveys, particularly from private sector institutions, were very low and "genomics" has many different meanings. Furthermore, the analysis of genomics R&D in the commercial sector is limited to publicly available data because few data are available about privately held firms. Despite these provisions, however, the data are probably the most comprehensive compiled to date and they suggest a number of important trends.

■ Private sector funding for genomics exceeds funding from public and not-for-profit organizations. In 2000, global public sector funding sources identified in the survey totalled just under US$ 2 billion, whereas R&D expenditure by the private sector was extrapolated to total at least US$ 3 billion (including dedicated genomics firms and genomics expenditure in large pharmaceutical companies, but not including R&D among almost 300 privately held "genomics" firms).

■ The majority of genomics funding, both public and private, is directed towards performers in the United States. Public funding for genomics in the USA vastly outstrips that in any other country (see Graph 1), and 71% of privately held genomics firms and 78% of publicly traded firms identified in the exercise are USA-based. While major pharmaceutical companies support genomics research in Europe and Asia, commercial activities are predominantly located in developed economies (with a few pockets of development in Brazil, China, India and elsewhere among developing economies).

■ The ownership of DNA patents and other intellectual property will be heavily focused in the United States. The explosion of DNA patents is shown in Graph 2. Over 80% of DNA patents granted by the US Patent and Trademark Office between 1980 and 1993 had a USA assignee.

The key inference is that the future profits and resource flows in genomics will be concentrated in the developed economies in general, and in the United States in particular, and driven by the health care markets of the developed world.

References:

1. World Survey of Funding for Genomics Research:
   http://www.stanford.edu/class/siw198q/websites/genomics/entry.htm
   (accessed February 12, 2002)

2. DNA Patent Database http://www.genomic.org (accessed February 12, 2002)

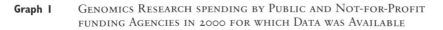

Graph 1 GENOMICS RESEARCH SPENDING BY PUBLIC AND NOT-FOR-PROFIT FUNDING AGENCIES IN 2000 FOR WHICH DATA WAS AVAILABLE

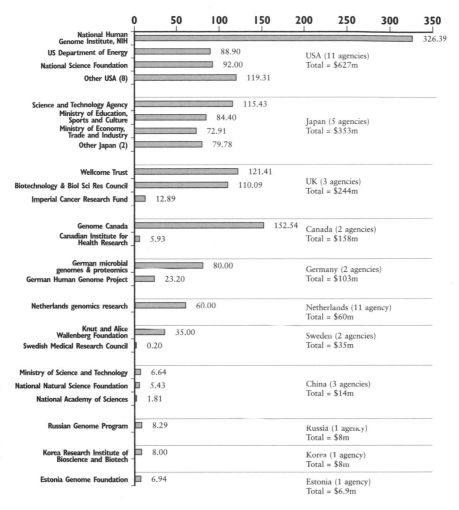

Source: World of Funding for Genomics Research: http://stanford.edu/class/siw198q/ websites/genomics/entry.htm

tries accounted for only 20% of the global pharmaceutical market, even though they made up over 80% of the world's population (Widdus, 2001).

Public research funding, on the other hand, could be directed by other considerations, including the need to narrow the developed-developing country gap, as opposed to commercial factors (see Section 5 for further discussion). In practice, however, public research programmes also tend to be focused on diseases such as cancer and cardiovascular diseases that are

Graph 2   DNA PATENTS GRANTED BY US PATENT OFFICE (1980–2000)

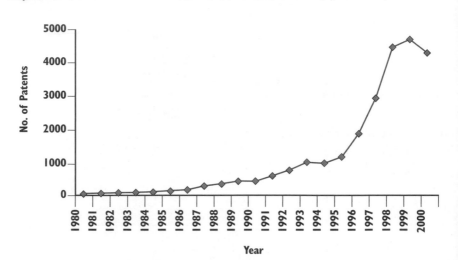

priorities in developed countries. Furthermore, public funding, both national and international, is in part driven by industrial concerns. For instance, many programmes supported by the European Community must include one or several industrial partners, thereby making it very difficult for projects which are not of interest to industry to obtain funding from this source.

Currently, therefore, the global research agenda appears to be determined largely by the markets in the developed countries, rather than the health needs of the developing world. It has been estimated, for example, that pneumonia, diarrhoea, tuberculosis and malaria, which together account for more than 20% of the disease burden of the world, receive less than 1% of the total public and private funds devoted to health research (Global Forum for Health Research, 2000). It was also estimated that in 1998, out of the US$ 70 billion global spending on health research, only US$ 300 million was directed to vaccines for HIV/AIDS and US$ 100 million to malarial research (UNDP, 2001).

As a result, the products of research are highly skewed in favour of the markets of the developed countries and to the detriment of developing country populations. For example, of the 1233 new drugs marketed between 1975 and 1999, only 13 were approved specifically for tropical diseases. Furthermore, of these, six were developed by WHO, United Nations Development Programme (UNDP) and UNDP/World

Bank/WHO-supported Special Programme for Research and Training in Tropical Diseases (TDR) (Pecoul et al., 1999).

7.3.2 Redressing the developed-developing country gap

The importance of increasing the technological capacity of the developing countries so that they can reap the health benefits from genomics, and some of the ways that this might be achieved, is outlined in Section 5.

The twin problems of how to redirect global resources into research and development that address the health priorities of developing countries, and how to make drugs and vaccines more accessible to developing country populations that need them, have been addressed in several international fora and reports. They also form the primary agenda of several international committees and organizations, including that of TDR, the Special Programme for Research, Development and Research Training in Human Reproduction (HRP) which is jointly sponsored by the UNDP, UNFPA, World Bank, WHO and the Global Forum for Health Research.

Since its inception in 1975, TDR has reported notable successes in its aim of directing research toward diseases of developing countries. In the context of genomics, it has been instrumental in establishing research networks for mapping the genomes of disease-causing parasites and ensuring that the data are freely accessible to other researchers. It is supporting research in genomics that will improve the understanding of tropical diseases, and lead to the identification of potential targets for drugs, vaccines, and diagnostics, as well as exploring the potential of using genetic modification of vectors as an approach to controlling infectious diseases.

In the 1980s, TDR became increasingly involved in working with commercial partners to take products for neglected diseases through to the development stage. Its interactions with the private sector have included the participation of scientists from the pharmaceutical industry in TDR's advisory committees, the provision of services to TDR from industry, and joint programmes with private companies. One outcome, for example, was the public-private partnership between WHO and Hoechst Marion Roussel Inc. which led to the production of eflornithine for the treatment of African trypanosomiasis. This success is an excellent model of public-private collaboration for the control of neglected diseases (Lucas, 2000).

While various commentators have been very positive regarding WHO participation in public-private partnerships, several have called for caution. For example, there is the possibility that WHO's normative functions could be subjected to commercial pressures. There is also the additional risk that WHO's primary concern with the most impoverished and hence least commercially attractive population groups could be subverted by the commercial concerns of its partners (Buse and Waxman, 2001).

Similar issues are also being addressed by the Global Forum for Health Research, an international foundation established to address the global imbalance in health research by improving the allocation of research funds and facilitating collaboration between the public and private sectors (Global Forum for Health Research, 2000). It supports the Initiative on Public-Private Partnerships, which reports that there are now more than 70 international public-private partnerships. Major examples include the International AIDS Vaccine Initiative, Global Alliance for TB Drug Development, and Medicines for Malaria Venture.

The Global Forum for Health Research organized the Global Health Forum I in February 2000 to discuss the strategy of using public-private partnerships in developing and delivering drugs and vaccines for neglected diseases. In its consensus statement (Global Health Forum I, 2000), four guiding principles are stated: first, the need for the public and private sectors to work in partnership at the global level; second, the need to use comprehensive approaches that encompass "push factors" such as subsidising the costs of research as well as "pull factors" such as establishing viable markets; third, the need to ensure that drugs and vaccines are delivered; and fourth, the need to sustain the momentum in achieving targets. Public-private initiatives, including drug donation and delivery programmes, were promoted as a method for accelerating the development of urgently needed drugs and improving access among those who are most in need.

Besides public-private partnerships, WHO has also approached the issue of differential pricing of essential drugs, that is for companies to charge different prices for drugs in different markets according to purchasing power. In a joint workshop with the World Trade Organization (WTO) in April 2001 (WHO and WTO Secretariats, 2001), these organizations brought together experts to consider differential pricing as a strategy for increasing access to essential drugs in developing countries. The conclusions reached affirm that differential pricing is a feasible strategy provided that certain conditions are met, including ways of preventing lower-priced drugs from reaching markets in developed countries. Corollary issues of voluntary licensing and generic drug production were also discussed as mechanisms that may be employed to increase competition and lower drug prices.

The need to channel resources into research that reflect the health priorities of developing countries is also addressed in other documents, among them the UNDP Human Development report (2001). This report focuses on how new technologies, including biotechnology, affect developing countries and deprived communities, the policies needed to prevent the exacerbation of existing inequalities, and the potential of harnessing the technologies to advance human development and eradicate poverty. It highlights the central place of genetics in medical sciences and the potential of genomics technologies. Nevertheless, it argues that the objective of eradicating poverty will not be achieved through the market, nor will national policies be sufficient to compensate for global market failures. Therefore, new international initiatives and the use of fair global rules are needed to channel novel technologies toward the urgent health needs of the world's poor. Examples given of mechanisms that might be used include dedicated funds for research and development, tax incentives, differential pricing, as well as fair use of intellectual property rights and implementation of the Trade-related Aspects of Intellectual Property Rights (TRIPS) Agreement (see Section 7.4.3). Finally, the report emphasizes the importance of using policy instruments to build technological capacity in developing countries. Interestingly, these approaches do not differ much from those suggested as a solution to the problem of the inadequate market barrier by the pharmaceutical industry (Sykes, 2000).

7.3.3   DEVELOPING RESEARCH CAPACITIES

While the future role of international organizations are important in steering global resources toward the health problems of developing countries, nevertheless, at the consultations that led up to this Report, it was emphasized that it is critical for developing countries, either individually or collectively, to begin now to develop research capacity in all areas of genomics, so that this technology can be applied to address local and regional health needs. While there probably will be some developments from genomics research conducted in the developed countries that will be applicable to developing countries, the latter cannot rely on the largely market-driven research agenda of the developed countries to address their health needs.

Some approaches to addressing this problem were outlined in Section 5. The strategy that each country adopts in developing research and development capacity will depend on its existing facilities and strengths. The coordination of research activity both at a national and a regional level will be critical for the effective application of genomics research. To enable developing countries to access technologies the development of regional partnerships will be particularly critical for countries which have only limited or minimal capacity at present. An appropriate model for building these partnerships might be to develop coordinated networks of collaborating research centres. Such networks could support effective exchange of information and avoid duplication of effort, both in terms of research and technology development, and could coordinate training activities and technology dissemination. It is essential that constituent centres each have a minimal level of scientific capability and a robust management structure. The system which is evolving in India is an approach of this kind which might be feasible in other countries (see Box 5.6).

The development of research partnerships with complementary expertise in the developed countries will also be crucial. In many cases, it will be cost-effective to utilize high throughput genomics technologies through such collaborations, rather than attempting to develop these highly expensive facilities in the short term. In the fields of genome sequencing and proteomics, there is a concern that developing countries may invest considerable funds in developing technology that would soon become obsolete. Careful consideration must therefore be given to the relative value of building this type of capacity as opposed to entering into partnerships with institutions in the developed countries.

As discussed in Section 5, whichever approach is taken it is essential that the problem of the loss of able scientists from the developing countries to the developed countries is addressed.

These organizational changes directed at improving the research and development capacities of the developing countries will undoubtedly require financial support. Recently, the Commission for Macroeconomics and Health was established by the Director-General of WHO for a period of two years to affirm the place of health in global economic development and with the ultimate goal of placing it at the top of the development agenda. One of the Commission's six working groups is also examining the issue of neglected diseases and the barriers for commercial research and development of preventive, diagnostic and therapeutic approaches to these diseases. The recommendations for research in the Commission's report (Commission on Macroeconomics and Health, 2001) are outlined in Section 4.4. Without an increased input of funding for research and development from the developed countries, as outlined in the Commission's report, there seems little doubt that any medical benefits which arise from research in genomics will simply widen the developed-developing country gap in research and development potential.

7.4 INTELLECTUAL PROPERTY AND SHARING THE BENEFITS OF RESEARCH

A recurrent theme that surfaced throughout the consultations prior to this Report was dissatisfaction with current intellectual property laws, their application to the patenting of genetic material, their interpretation in the context of access to drugs and international trade agreements, and the impact on public health in developing countries. The problems surrounding intellectual property and international trade agreements are complex, interlocking, and contentious. This Section provides an outline of the major issues as a preliminary step for considering WHO's approach to these problems.

7.4.1 Patents

Patents are awarded for inventions, granting monopolies to inventors for a limited period of time in exchange for public disclosure of the invention. The temporary monopoly allows the inventor to earn profits without having to face competition if the invention is commercialized, thereby rewarding the inventor and encouraging innovation.

Generally, patents are only awarded if an invention can meet three criteria, novelty, inventiveness and utility. Novelty requires that the invention is not known prior to the patent application, while utility requires that the invention is useful, or has industrial applicability. The invention also has to incorporate an inventive step, that is, it should not be obvious to a person with ordinary skill in the relevant field. The disclosure criteria requires that the invention is developed and explained in a way that allows a person with ordinary skills in the relevant field to utilize it.

There are different types of patents: product patents, which cover pharmacologically active chemicals or formulations; process patents, covering a manufacturing process for a product; and use patents, covering the use of a product. A product covered by a product patent may not be produced without licence even if a different method is used to produce it, but a process patent does not prohibit a third party from manufacturing the product without licence if a different method is used.

Patents are based on national or regional legislation, which varies widely in terms of what may be patented, the criteria that have to be met, the methods by which the application is assessed, and the terms and conditions under which patents are awarded. Disclosure criteria may also vary. The process from patent application to the patent being issued may take a few years, and the patent applicant has to bear the costs of application as well as its legal protection in case of subsequent litigation.

7.4.2   Patenting genetic material

Many thousands of patents with claims to human DNA sequences have been filed and granted. These include genomic DNA sequences, SNPs (see Section 2), DNA sequences of individual mutations that give rise to diseases, cloning vectors, proteins or parts of proteins, and computer-assisted methods for identifying proteins or parts of proteins of similar structure. In a few cases patented sequences have been approved for gene-based diagnostic tests, for example, cystic fibrosis and breast cancer. Due of differences in policies regarding the patenting of DNA (Box 7.2), more patents of this kind have been filed in the United States than in other parts of the world.

Currently, the situation regarding the patenting of discoveries arising from genomics is little less than chaotic and has come under fierce criticism from many quarters (Bobrow and Thomas, 2001; Williamson, 2001). It is argued that a normal or abnormal gene sequence is, in effect, naturally occurring information which cannot therefore be patentable. The counter-argument which has been used widely by patent lawyers, that DNA sequence identification is a form of purification "outside the body," and therefore analogous to the purification of naturally occurring pharmacological agents, is specious; the DNA molecule is not, in this context, important as a substance and its value resides in its information content. Similar arguments have been used for patenting complementary DNA sequences (cDNAs), that is DNA synthesized on a messenger RNA template, which has no introns (i.e. sequences of DNA that are not ultimately translated into the final protein, see Section 2). This is based on the notion that a "natural" gene contains introns, and therefore synthesizing complementary DNA is an "alteration" of nature and as such amounts to a human invention. However, as pointed out by Bobrow and Thomas (2001) messenger RNA exists in nature, and cDNA is just a translation of this sequence. In other words it is rather like saying that the same invention could be repatented if translated into a different language.

However, despite the fact that DNA sequences represent naturally occurring information patents continue to be granted. Although the US Constitution (Box 7.2) allows discoveries as well as inventions, in current

Box 7.2 THE USA AND EUROPEAN PATENT SYSTEMS AND THE PATENTING OF GENOMIC INFORMATION

Both the United States Patent and Trademark Office (USPTO) and the European Patent Office (EPO) require that for a patent to be granted on a particular invention it must meet three criteria, namely that it must be novel, it must involve an inventive step and it must have a demonstrated "utility" or clear industrial applicability. Although the US constitution does provide for the granting of patents on discoveries, current practice requires that the patent application must include an inventive step above that involved in a discovery of something that exists in nature. There are a number of key differences between the USA and European patent systems in terms of current patenting processes as shown in the table below.

Patents with broad claims are being granted on genes, predominantly by the USPTO. It is important to note that a patent cannot be granted on a gene as it occurs naturally. Current practice requires isolation of the gene, and the precedent cited is purification of a natural product. The patent offices have elected to treat each new gene as a new chemical compound and grant "composition of matter" patents. The USPTO adopts the position that however obvious the method of isolation of a gene, the sequence is not obvious and on this basis, such a patent is justified. In January 2001, the USPTO published revised utility examination guidelines, stressing that a patent application must disclose a "specific, substantial and credible utility for the claimed isolated and purified gene." Williamson (2001) points out that the USPTO will still accept an electronic comparison with a structural analogue as the basis for utility, even though this contradicts its own criterion for obviousness.

The patenting of gene sequences has been less readily accepted in Europe so far. However, the 1998 European Parliament Directive on the Legal Protection of Biotechnological Inventions (The EU Biotechnology Directive – 98/44/EC) does allow for the patenting of whole or partial gene sequences. Article 5 of the legislation states that "An element isolated from the human body or otherwise produced by means of a technical process, including the sequence or partial sequence of a gene, may constitute a patentable invention, even if the structure of that element is identical to that of a natural element" This legislation, which underwent a protracted preparation process lasting 10 years, has been challenged by a number of EU Member States.

Comparison of United States and European Patent Office Protocols (based on Williamson 2001)

United States Patent and Trademark Office (USPTO)	European Patent Office) (EPO
A patent is awarded to the *first to invent* in cases of duplication	A patent is awarded to the *first to file* in cases of duplication
The inventor has a 12-month grace period during which he can publish the invention and improve upon it without compromising the invention.	No grace period
The patent application is published 18 months after the filing date*	The patent application is published 18 months after the filing date

Box 7.2 (CONTINUED)

United States Patent and Trademark Office (USPTO)	European Patent Office) (EPO
The patent is valid for 20 years	The patent is valid for 20 years
There is no opposition mechanism within the patent office. Legal tests of patents occur in the courts	An opposition can be brought to the EPO within nine months of the patent being granted

NB: Until November 2000 when USPTO changed its publication practice to reflect that in Europe, patents were not published until they were granted

References

1. Williamson AR (2001). Gene patents: socially acceptable monopolies or an unnecessary hindrance to research?. Trends in Genetics, 17: 670–673.

2. United States Federal Register (2001). Utility Examination Guidelines, 5th January. *United States Federal Register* 66(4):1092–1099.

3. Directive 98/44/EC of the European Parliament and of the Council of 6 July 1998 on the legal protection of biotechnological inventions (398L0044) *Official Journal L 213, 30/07/1998 p. 0013–0021*

practice patents are not supposed to be allowed on discovery. For a patent to be granted in either Europe or the USA, an invention must be novel, show utility, and be capable of industrial application. In practice, however, these criteria do not seem to be met in many cases.

It has been concluded that on balance, the current position regarding DNA patenting is retarding rather than stimulating both scientific and economic progress. The monopolies awarded by patents on genes as novel chemicals are not therefore in the public interest (Williamson, 2001) and, as pointed out by Barton (2001), this unsatisfactory situation has important implications for the health of the developing countries. In essence, it weakens the contribution of the global research community to the creation and application of medical technology for these countries, and, in the long-term, may complicate the granting of concessional prices for therapeutic agents. In addition, there are already signs that the position regarding the patenting of proteins, more important products for generating these agents, is becoming even more chaotic than DNA patenting (Service, 2001).

Numerous international bodies and policy-makers have made statements directed at the reform of the patent system (Box 7.3) but this has not led to a coherent policy framework. The attention of policy-makers has been uneven and there have been few attempts to grapple with the patent system as a whole.

Box 7.3 Positions of International Organizations on Patenting of the Genome

As the Human Genome Project enters its final stages, a number of international organizations have asserted the need to ensure that these data are made freely available in the public domain and expressed their concerns regarding current trends in intellectual property. Despite these representations, there has been little progress in harmonizing these issues.

International Statements

In March, 2000, USA President, Bill Clinton, and United Kingdom Prime Minister, Tony Blair released a joint statement asserting that "to realize the full potential of this [human genome] research, raw fundamental data on the human genome... should be made freely available to scientists everywhere." The statement goes on to affirm that "gene-based inventions will also play an important role in stimulating the development of important new health care products."

In July 2000, the G8 Summit's Okinawa Communique called for "the further rapid release of all raw fundamental data on human DNA sequences" and emphasizes the "importance of pursuing the postgenome sequence research on the basis of multilateral collaboration."

The United Nations Millennial Declaration (September 2000) resolves "to ensure free access to information on the human genome sequence."

The Human Genome Organization (HUGO)

The role of HUGO as the coordinating body for the international Human Genome Project was affirmed at the First International Strategy Meeting on Human Genome Sequencing (Bermuda, 1996) at which partners in the Human Genome Project resolved that primary genomic sequence should be in the public domain and rapidly released. HUGO has released two statements on gene patenting — the first in 1995, and an updated statement in April 2000 in response to the European Biotechnology Directive and other developments. The latter stresses the need for patent authorities to require "unambiguous indication and enabling disclosure of function" for claimed DNA molecules, and asserts that single nucleotide polymorphisms (SNPs) "cannot as a rule meet the requirements of inventiveness." It also released a statement on the Early Release of Raw Sequence data in 1997 which urges patent offices to rescind decisions to grant patents on expressed sequence tags (ESTs) as probes to identify specific DNA sequences.

UNESCO

Article 4 of the Universal Declaration on the Human Genome and Human Rights, which was adopted by the UNESCO General Assembly in 1998, states that "the human genome in its natural state shall not give rise to financial gains." The International Bioethics Committee (IBC) of UNESCO is responsible for promoting the principles detailed in the Universal Declaration, and hence has a major interest in the patenting debate. In January 2001, UNESCO hosted an international symposium on Ethics, Intellectual Property and Genomics, at which participants from all sides of the gene patenting debate discussed the issues of contention. Participants highlighted existing ambiguities in existing legal provisions on patenting which will be difficult to harmonize and concerns that current practices will impede research in developing countries. The IBC convened a working group to examine the issues raised at the meeting, which reported to the eighth session of the IBC in September 2001. As a result the IBC released a position statement stating that "there

---

Box 7.3 (CONTINUED)

was strong ethical grounds for excluding the human genome from patentability," and that this principle should be adopted in the revision of the TRIPS agreement.

Other Organizations

The Council of Europe has proposed to develop a code of conduct that guarantees both free scientific access to genetic resources as well as the sharing of ensuing benefits with developing countries. The European Forum of Medical Associations and the WHO European Regional Office have released a statement asserting that the ethical and moral problems associated with the granting of patents on the human genome and its sequences should be debated by the public, politicians and the scientific community.

Further Information

1. Human Genome Organization website: http://www.gene.ucl.ac.uk/hugo/
2. UNESCO Bioethics website: http://www.unesco.org/ibc/
3. Council of Europe:
   http://www.coe.int
4. G8 Okinawa Communique: http://www.mofa.go.jp/policy/economy/summit/2000/documents/communique.html
5. United Nations Millennial Declaration: http://www.un.org/millennium/
6. World Health Organization Regional Office for Europe (2001). *European Forum for Medical Associations and WHO: report on a WHO meeting, Warsaw, Poland, 17–19 March, 2000.* Copenhagen, WHO Regional Office for Europe. EUR/00/5016633/5. http://www.who.dk/document/e71875.pdf

---

Clearly there needs to be a very clear articulation and discussion of certain key questions (Bobrow and Thomas, 2001); can patents on DNA sequences continue to be justified in the context of current technology? Are such patents really necessary for successful innovation in health care? What are the real thresholds for novelty, inventiveness and utility? What are the duties of patent holders in licensing their inventions? These problems need to be addressed by an international policy forum, a role for which WHO is ideally suited. If some sense is not made of this complex and chaotic situation quickly, both the biomedical research community and industry will be severely disadvantaged in their efforts to translate the potential of genomics into improvements of global health. It is vital, therefore, that strong international leadership is directed at finding a solution to these problems which, if not solved, will undoubtedly exacerbate further the discrepancies between the provision of health care among the different countries of the world.

7.4.3   The TRIPS agreement

In 1995, the Marrakech Agreement established the World Trade Organization (WTO), an international body to deal with the rules of trade among nations, with the objective of setting in place a multilateral trading system by liberalizing trading policies throughout the world. The WTO has 142 member countries (as of 26 July 2001), and the ministerial conference is the highest level decision-making body.

In the WTO, countries negotiate and draw up agreements which bind them to the way in which their trade will be conducted. One of these agreements, the Trade-related Aspects of Intellectual Property Rights (TRIPS) agreement (1994), establishes minimum standards on intellectual property by which member countries have to abide by specified deadlines. Developed countries had to amend their respective patent acts to conform with the TRIPS standards by 1996, developing countries by 2000, and least developed countries by 2006.

Under TRIPS, patent protection had to be provided for a period of no less than 20 years, and had to be extended equally to all patented products, whether imported or locally produced. TRIPS required the patentability of microorganisms and of nonbiological and microbiological processes for the production of plants and animals as well as pharmaceuticals. However, it allowed the following to be excluded from patentability: diagnostic, therapeutic, and surgical methods and procedures for the treatment of humans and other animals, of plants and animals other than microorganisms, and of natural biological processes for the production of plants and animals.

Although the TRIPS agreement permits countries to licence the production of cheaper copies of patented drugs where this is necessary on public health grounds, if all its members had to recognize patents by 2006, as originally planned, these rights would have been lost. However, in a declaration agreed at the WTO meeting in Doha, Qatar, in November 2001 (World Trade Organization, 2001), this deadline was postponed to 2016 for least-developed countries. Furthermore, it states that the agreement should be implemented in a manner that is "supportive of WTO members' rights to protect public health and in particular to promote access to medicines for all." In addition, individual countries will be free to determine the circumstances under which licences to manufacture generics are issued. The declaration also acknowledges that these are not confined to emergency situations, but if countries declare an emergency they can issue compulsory licences without prior negotiation with the patent owner (Cherry, 2001).

Clearly, the recent declaration made in Doha, Qatar is a step in the right direction for protecting the health interests of the developing countries. However, TRIPS does not contain any explicit references to genetic material, and this provides another reason why WHO needs to take a major lead in the rationalisation of the current situation regarding the patenting of the products of genomics research.

7.4.4   Biological resources and benefit sharing

The developing countries are a rich source of genetic biodiversity, and their populations often have knowledge of how to identify plants and animals that have medicinal or other uses. Through the years, collections of biological specimens or the genetic material extracted from these sources have sometimes been transported to the developed countries. Furthermore, traditional knowledge about the uses of such materials is usually in the public domain, and in many cases has been systematically recorded by researchers.

Bioprospecting, or the search for useful genes and biochemicals from among the biological resources of countries, continues to be carried out by researchers from academic and government institutions, as well as private companies. While much of this work is directed at studies of population genetics or disease mechanisms, increasingly the purpose is primarily to find genetic material that can be used to develop pharmaceutical, agricultural, or other useful products that could then be patented and marketed for profit. The concern is that developing countries, as the suppliers of genetic material, may end up having to pay high prices for the products that are eventually developed from these materials.

Most controversies in this field have been over plant genetic material and its derivatives. Several patents have been sought by developed countries on plants and crops of the developing world, for example neem, basmati rice and Mexican yellow beans, resulting in strong protests. In late 2001, a conflict erupted between farmers, civil society groups and agricultural authorities in Thailand, and an American researcher who was attempting to produce a mutant form of jasmine rice that could be grown in the USA. The Thai authorities accused the research worker of obtaining the genetic material of the rice without permission. This case highlights the concerns of developing countries that such practices will endanger both exports and the livelihood of traditional farmers.

In addition, patents filed on DNA or cell lines of indigenous peoples are raising increasing concerns. As well as the potential exploitation of this material, this trend is having the unfortunate effect of generating increased opposition to vital population genetic studies and other work of direct medical benefit to many countries.

Benefit sharing has been proposed as a solution to these problems. One of the three objectives of the Convention on Biological Diversity (CBD) is the fair and equitable sharing of benefits arising from the utilization of genetic resources (CBD, Article 1). The Conference of Parties, the governing body of the CBD, addressed this issue for the first time as a main item of its fourth meeting (May 1998). Since then, it has convened the Panel of Experts on Access and Benefit Sharing to conduct further work on this issue, and also established an Ad Hoc Open-ended Working Group with the mandate to develop guidelines and other approaches for submission to the Conference of Parties at its sixth meeting, and to assist countries and stakeholders in various aspects of benefit sharing. The CBD web site is currently collecting case studies of benefit sharing from all around the world. Although the CBD highlights the need for benefit sharing with local and indigenous communities, it does not provide legal rights to local communities regarding their knowledge or genetic resources; legislation is left to national governments.

An approach to benefit sharing that has been incorporated into national and regional legislation is exemplified in the Common System on Access to Genetic Resources (referred to as Common System), adopted by the Andean Pact (Dutfield, 2001). The latter is a customs union agreed at Cartagena, Colombia (therefore sometimes also known as the Cartagena Agreement) in 1969 among five countries: Bolivia, Chile, Colombia, Ecuador and Peru. Venezuela joined the union, but Chile left, in 1976. In 1996, the Andean Pact countries adopted the Common System which establishes region-wide access and benefit sharing regimes. The Common System states that member countries have sovereign rights over the use and exploitation of their genetic resources, including derivatives of these resources, and the right to determine conditions of access. It also extends rights over an "intangible component," which refers to any knowledge, innovation or practice associated with a biogenetic resource or its derivative. Under this system, researchers who access genetic resources in these countries are required to sign an access contract before the research is carried out. These contracts have to take into account the rights and interests of the suppliers of genetic resources, and their derivatives and related intangible components, and guarantee the equitable sharing of benefits derived from access to these resources.

The Andean Pact was brought in line with TRIPS with the adoption of Decision 486 on December 1, 2000, under which patenting of microorganisms was introduced. Nevertheless, TRIPS does not recognize the contribution of traditional knowledge, or the need for benefit sharing. There have been proposals that provisions for incorporating benefit sharing concerns are explicitly written into TRIPS to protect traditional knowledge and genetic resources. Further discussion needs to be developed at the WTO on this issue.

The Human Genome Organization (HUGO) Ethics Committee statement on benefit sharing (HUGO, 2000) considers these issues as applied to genetic research conducted among human populations. It sets out some general principles, including the necessity for prior consultation with participating individuals and communities, during which issues related to affordability and accessibility of eventual products of research should be discussed. It recommends that benefits are not limited to individuals who participate in the research but that profit-making entities dedicate a percentage, for example from 1% to 3% of their annual net profits, to health care infrastructure and humanitarian efforts for the community.

Among other organizations, the United States National Bioethics Advisory Commission also recommends that prior agreements are forged between research sponsors and local representatives, so that countries can set their own priorities for research that is undertaken, based on the potential benefit that will be fed back to the community. The International Bioethics Committee of UNESCO has supported the idea of benefit sharing (UNESCO, 2001) and recognized the need for global benefit sharing agreements and the development of novel mechanisms of intellectual property management that uphold the public good.

As genomic research expands, the possibilities for work involving the resources of the developing countries will undoubtedly increase. Although some progress has been made towards the definition of benefit sharing, a great deal more work is required, particularly to ensure that international research collaborations are based on benefit sharing programmes which do not have potential disadvantages for the health and economy of the developing countries.

7.5   OWNERSHIP AND ACCESS TO GENETIC DATABASES

The rationale and potential hazards of the increasing development of large genetic databases were outlined in Section 6 and some of the ethical issues which are posed by this new trend in genomics research are discussed in Section 8.

As pointed out in Section 6, in the case of some of the very large population databases that are being developed, although there is some provision for repatriation of any profits that accrue to the community this is not always the case. For example, it is far from clear whether the people who donate their genetic material and information in the very large United Kingdom database will share any possible benefits that arise (United Kingdom House of Lords Select Committee on Science and Technology, 2001).

Indeed, the economic issues relating to the ownership, benefits accrual, and access to genetic databases for research are subjects of contention. It has been argued that if it is the expressed purpose of a piece of research to develop profitable new drugs, then it is not unreasonable for individuals who allow access to their DNA to consider themselves as owners of a resource and to demand fair compensation, which is considered to be in the region of 50% of net profits and royalties (Bear, 2001). It is further argued that although there is ethical objection to making a profit from genetic material, nevertheless, human DNA is in reality commercialized, and as such, appropriate compensation for individuals in exchange for commercial access to their DNA is in line with respect for human rights. Although this argument is essentially for individual benefit, it is also suggested that governments which mediate between commercial interests and their population's DNA should estimate appropriate level access fees. This would greatly exceed current levels of returns to donors of genetic information, including the 1–3% of net profits recommended by the HUGO Ethics Committee.

Each national government will have to consider these issues in relation to the interests of its peoples. Nevertheless, genomic and pharmaceutical companies may have more expertise and experience in negotiation than the governments of developing countries. There is a need therefore for countries to acquire the capacity to carry out such negotiations. WHO may therefore consider a role in convening fora among various stakeholders to discuss these issues, establishing international guidelines, and helping governments to clarify the issues and develop the expertise and skill needed to negotiate with multinational companies.

7.6   Summary

Fears that the unequal distribution of the potential medical benefits which may be generated by genomics research could exacerbate current inequalities in the provision of health care among nations are well-founded. Although some progress is being made towards improving the situation, many problems remain, particularly in the areas of infrastructure, biotechnological development, patenting DNA, benefit sharing, and the commercial implications of large population data collections.

8. ETHICAL ISSUES IN GENETIC RESEARCH, SCREENING, AND TESTING, WITH PARTICULAR REFERENCE TO DEVELOPING COUNTRIES

Contents

8.1   INTRODUCTION

The coming genomics era will raise important ethical issues and challenges. These can and should be addressed in a manner that will allow the health benefits of this new era to be realized. Most of the ethical issues raised by genomics for developing countries are not new, but are found in other areas of biology and medicine. In particular, many of those discussed below, such as informed consent, confidentiality, and stigmatization and discrimination, are not unique to genomics. Nevertheless, even these familiar ethical issues require some specific consideration in the context of genomics and cannot simply be addressed by standard approaches in medical ethics for two reasons.

First, genetic information and potential genetic interventions are different in some important respects from most medical and health information and interventions, in many cases in degree and in others in kind. For example, since genetic information about individuals can be highly predictive of their future health, it has the potential both to stigmatize them and to be used by others such as potential employers and insurers as a basis for discrimination. These issues provide grounds for strong confidentiality protections. In the different context of families, however, there may be reasons to put special limits on confidentiality, since genetic information about an individual is often equally relevant to his or her family members. In the reproductive context, interventions to prevent genetic transmission of serious disease to children often involve abortion which does not simply prevent the disease, as in other branches of preventive medicine, but prevents the birth of a child who would have the disease. At some point in the future it may become possible to manipulate the genetic inheritance of children not just to prevent disease, but to enhance normal functions. Both of these latter kinds of interventions are condemned by some as eugenic and will be addressed later in this section. The history of eugenics in the late 19th and the first half of the 20th centuries more generally casts a shadow over modern genomics and contributes to widespread unease over our expanding potential for genetic control of human nature.

The second reason why these ethical issues require distinct treatment here is the importance of the social context in which the issues arise; in particular, they may be significantly different in developing than in developed countries, as well as among different developing countries. The importance of this point cannot be over-emphasized. The appropriate uses of our new genetic knowledge and capacities, the potential for their misuse or abuse, as well as the kinds of responses needed to prevent such misuse or abuse, all depend critically on social, political, economic and cultural contexts. By way of illustration, in countries without strong cultural and legal traditions of respecting individual reproductive freedom, the potential for coercion of women's reproductive choices for eugenic or other reasons is magnified. In highly patriarchal societies where men traditionally make important decisions for family members, including their wives, women are again especially vulnerable to coercion in making reproductive choices and it will be more difficult to ensure their free and informed consent for genetic services. In countries with significant private health insurance, there is a potential for genetic discrimination by insurers that will not exist in those with a national health service available to all. The populations of very poor developing countries are especially vulnerable to economic exploitation by much richer developed countries or multinational corporations in genetic research or the development and use of genetic databases. Finally, low education levels in some developing countries and limited familiarity with genetic medicine or research present special obstacles to obtaining truly informed consent from the population.

A general feature of many developing countries is a lack of any well-developed regulatory apparatus to deal with either the scientific issues in genetic research and technology, or with the ethical, legal, and social issues (see Section 6). An important priority for many developing countries as genomics becomes more prominent in them should be to develop the necessary regulatory structures to address both the scientific and ethical issues. In some cases broad international guidelines should be created to help to guide the development of genomics and of country-specific guidelines in developing and developed countries. Some of this guideline development has already been done, but much remains to be done and WHO has an opportunity to play a leadership role here.

This Section begins by discussing two central ethical issues that any country should address before engaging in genetic research or initiating genetic screening and testing programmes: informed consent and confidentiality of genetic information to prevent discrimination and stigmatization.

8.2   INFORMED CONSENT

8.2.1   *Principles*

As a result of past abuses of research participants in many countries, the principle that subjects cannot be enrolled in research without their free and informed consent is well-established in international documents such as the Nuremberg principles and the Declaration of Helsinki, in the law of many countries, as well as in research practice. Unlike medical therapy where the goal is the patient's well being, the goal of research is generalizable knowledge and so there is a potential conflict of interest between the researcher and the research subject (Faden and Beauchamp, 1986). This warrants giving special importance to the informed consent of a potential subject. Genetic research involving human subjects is no different. The consent process employed when developed-country researchers undertake research in developing countries should be sensitive and responsive to local cultural and social beliefs and practices, and it should not violate international standards nor be one that would be ethically unacceptable in their own countries.

The principle, and even more the practice, of informed consent in medical therapy is less well-established and respected than in medical research in both some developed and developing countries. Paternalistic traditions in the medical profession, where it is assumed that physicians are acting for the welfare of their patients, are still powerful in many countries and result in inadequate informed consent practices. Nevertheless, it is increasingly widely recognized that competent patients should not receive either diagnostic or therapeutic interventions without their free and informed consent. Respecting patients' rights to give or withhold consent respects their self-determination and their right to bodily integrity. When countries implement genetic screening programmes, which by definition are directed at a specific population, individuals should not be included in these programmes without having given their free and informed consent. Even when the screening is only to establish epidemiological data, the informed consent of participants must be obtained.

In some cultural contexts that lack any strong tradition or practice of individual consent, it may be more common for community leaders to give consent for screening or research programmes in their community. While it is appropriate to respect these cultural practices and to seek the agreement of properly identified community leaders to undertake screening or research programmes, it should not substitute for securing the consent of individual participants as well. Research projects in developed countries typically require written consent, but in cultures in which there is reluctance for a variety of reasons to sign a written document, oral consent can substitute for written consent, as it often does for medical therapy that does not carry high risks.

8.2.2   Genetic testing in health care and research

Genetic testing is typically targeted at particular individuals at risk for specific disease. As in medical research, medical therapy, and genetic screening, it too should not be undertaken without first securing the individual's free and informed consent. The consent process should include pre-test genetic counselling concerning the condition being tested for, which should be followed by post-test counselling (Nuffield Council on Bioethics, 1993). This counselling is especially important when the level of understanding of genetics and its role in disease is low, yet capacities for high-quality genetic counselling are strained even in developed countries, and are extremely limited in many developing countries. As countries introduce genetic testing programmes, they should simultaneously build capacities for high-quality genetic counseling.

Experience in a number of countries has already demonstrated the potential for coercive pressures from government, society, or family members in genetic screening and testing programmes. For example, in some countries it is now mandatory to have a test for thalassaemia before getting married. While couples are often not pressured to act on the information, in some cases pressure is brought to bear. Health authorities may perceive that prenatal diagnosis for a disease like thalassaemia is effective and much cheaper than treating a child with regular blood transfusions for 20 or 30 years; consequently, pressure may be put on couples to undergo testing and to avoid marriage or terminate a pregnancy when necessary.

Coercive social pressures can also come from potential stigmatization of parents for not using genetic testing. For example, in some countries in which there is a high take up of prenatal diagnosis of thalassaemia, even in apparent absence of explicit pressure put on couples, those who decline testing and have a child with thalassaemia may be strongly stigmatized for doing so. Even when there are strong ethical reasons to prevent the birth of children with serious genetically transmitted diseases, respecting individuals' human right to reproductive freedom requires leaving them free to make their own informed choices. However, these coercive pressures on reproductive choices can be subtle and are often extremely difficult to prevent. Both regulatory and long-term education efforts will be needed to counter them.

When genetic testing services are not a part of universal health services, but instead are available only to those who can pay for them with private funds, the clearly inequitable result could be a concentration of genetically transmitted diseases among the poor in society; this would exacerbate inequalities in those societies by creating a genetic, as well as social and economic, underclass. When genetic testing and screening programmes are introduced in a country, they should be made a part of the universal health care services, available to all and not only in the private health sector where they will worsen health and other inequities.

There are several reasons why informed consent for genetic research, screening, and testing often has special importance in many developing countries. First, in many cases genetic tests are developed before any effective therapeutic intervention exists for those found to have a genetic risk. It is then especially important that individuals understand this fact as well as the potential longer-term psychological, emotional, and social consequences of learning of genetic risks in the absence of therapeutic means for eliminating them. This information can have profound effects on individuals' sense of identity and conceptions of themselves as healthy or diseased. There is also a potential for social misallocation of health resources if genetic tests come into wide use in the absence of cost-effective therapeutic interventions necessary to produce health gains for the population tested.

Second, when educational levels are relatively low and potential research subjects have limited familiarity with medical research, the informed consent process is essential so that they can have an adequate understanding of the research and their potential role in it before deciding whether to participate. In the case of genetic screening or testing, low educational levels in many developing countries mean that many potential participants will be relatively uninformed about the nature of the condition being screened or tested for, as well as about the possible implications and uses, both positive and negative, of the information obtained. This places special obligations on investigators or those carrying out genetic screening or testing to ensure that information is provided in a form that is understandable to participants, and appropriate to their educational levels and cultural context. Research is needed, in both developed and developing countries, about how best to provide relevant information.

Third, when only limited medical care is available in a country, participation in research may be the only effective means of obtaining it, creating coercive pressures to participate in the research. Especially in very poor countries, financial incentives to participate in research may also create undue pressures to participate.

Fourth, those performing genetic research in developing countries are often scientists from developed countries or large multinational pharmaceutical or biotechnology companies with research agendas different from the needs of developing countries. Substantial international consensus has developed that research should not be done in developing countries that does not have potential benefits for their populations. Genetic and other research in developing countries should be directed at health problems in those countries. To avoid exploitation, there must be reasonable assurance that the benefits of the research will be available at least to the research participants, and to the broader community in which the research is completed. There is considerable debate about what precisely this "reasonable assurance" responsibility requires; for example, what interventions must be available, from whom, to whom, for how long?, and so forth. The means by which this responsibility will be carried out should be worked out between investigators and representatives of the community in which the research will be done prior to commencement of the research, and should be detailed in the initial informed consent process. In general, there is a high potential for exploitation of relatively poor and uneducated members of developing countries by outside organizations and corporations whose primary mission is not the health of members of those countries; a meaningful informed consent process is one means of protecting against such exploitation. Some ways in which this complex issue might be addressed are discussed in Section 7.4.4.

8.2.3   Other approaches to regulating genetic testing, screening and research

The informed consent process should not be the only means of regulating and controlling genetic research or the use of genetic screening and testing, however, especially in developing countries. Health ministries should develop formal structures for the evaluation of potential genetic screening, research or testing programmes to ensure that the programmes address local health needs in a cost-effective manner. These regulatory structures should also be charged with addressing, on an ongoing basis, the ethical, legal and social implications (ELSI) of genetic screening, research and testing programmes in the country, including the development of appropriate regulations.

Diseases whose cause is largely genetic represent increasing proportions of the disease burden in many developing countries, especially in those in which malnutrition and communicable disease are coming under control. In such cases genetic screening, research or testing focused on those diseases particularly prevalent in the area will often be a cost-effective use of public health resources. In less advanced developing countries where public health and health care resources are extremely limited, other resource uses directed at communicable diseases and basic public health measures may often have greater priority than most or all genetic services. Countries should not leave the introduction of genetic testing programmes to the private sector where profit potential may be the primary motivation and the testing may not represent a good use of limited health resources.

8.2.4   Genetic databases

Another form of genetic research in some countries is the development of health information databases (see Section 6.5). Some developing countries, or geographical areas within developing countries, represent desirable opportunities for the development of such databases when the population is relatively genetically homogenous from limited migration in or out of the area and from founder effects. These databases vary in the extent to which data in them remain individually identifiable, though individual data are typically made non-identifiable to users of the database.

The databases are in some cases developed by public health authorities in the country, sometimes in partnership with private corporations as in the deCODE database in Iceland (Gulcher and Stefansson, 2000), and in other cases predominantly by private corporations. These databases raise a number of ethical issues, including profit sharing with the community from which the data are gathered (see Section 6), but here we focus on informed consent from individuals whose health information is placed in the database.

One central point of debate in the Icelandic project has been whether to employ an "opt-in" consent process, whereby individuals must explicitly consent to information about them being put in the database, or an "opt-out" process where, unless individuals object to information about them being entered into the database, the information will be included. In general, opt-out informed consent processes are not considered adequate for either medical research or therapy. Individuals should have to make a free and informed choice to participate before researchers can enroll them or before therapists can treat them.

In the Icelandic case, supporters of the opt-out consent process have relied mainly on the argument that data will only be drawn from existing medical records, no new genetic information will be gathered from individuals, and data will not be individually identifiable to the users of the database; data will be processed through a double encryption process. Of course, non-identifiability of participants in itself is not sufficient to justify opt-out consent since the results of most research are presented in a form in which individual participants are not identifiable. The database project in Iceland has generated some controversy, but seems to have strong public support and will be under the control of the Icelandic Government, who will grant an exclusive license to a private corporation to operate the database.

Presumed consent with an opt-out procedure should be adopted only with great caution and in special cases, since it is essentially the abandonment of the requirement that individuals must give their free and informed consent for research participation. Presumed consent is not a form of consent, as are written and oral consent, but rather represents a policy that individual consent is not necessary and that individuals will be included in the project unless they explicitly object.

A second important informed consent issue, both for databases and for other genetic research is whether health information or genetic material can be used for other purposes beyond those for which consent was originally given without obtaining additional consent for the new uses. As a general principle, uses of genetic material or information should not extend beyond those for which consent has been given. This problem is best dealt with at the time of the initial consent by specifying clearly the uses for which consent is given; in some cases the consent may be relatively open-ended, permitting as yet unanticipated uses in the future. But if consent is given only for specific and limited uses, then subjects should be recontacted and their consent obtained for any new uses of their genetic material or information.

8.3 CONFIDENTIALITY OF GENETIC INFORMATION TO PREVENT DISCRIMINATION AND STIGMATIZATION

8.3.1 *Confidentiality and its appropriate limits*

As genetics becomes increasingly integrated into clinical medicine, reproductive decision-making and public health, genetic information will accumulate about the genomes of individuals and groups. This information will often have a far-reaching impact on the individuals and groups in question, and if they are to cooperate freely in the development and use of this information they should have assurance about how the information will be used and who will have access to it (Rothstein, 1997).

Of course, even before the advent of modern genetics, health care systems have faced these issues with other non-genetic health care information about individuals or groups, including information about family history that often had similar predictive import to that of genetic information. In most countries such information is properly treated as confidential and not to be released to others without the patient's consent, although it can be released in therapeutic contexts on a "need to know" basis to others involved in the care of the patient. The legal and professional protections of the confidentiality of health care information vary from country to country and reflect cultural differences, but there is general international consensus on the practice of confidentiality. Does the prospect of increased genetic information pose any new ethical issues about confidentiality for health care and other systems in which that information will exist, in particular in developing countries?

One respect in which genetic information is different than other health care information, in degree if not in kind, is that it is typically not just about a particular individual who has been screened or tested, but also involves other family members of that individual. Genetic information about a specific health or reproductive risk of a particular individual will often imply a similar risk for other family members. In cases of relatively isolated groups which are unusually genetically homogenous, information about individuals may have implications about the wider group, not just other immediate family members. Second, genetic information is commonly predictive of an individual's risk of developing certain diseases in the future. Sometimes the condition can be predicted with a high degree of certainty, such as with the thalassaemias, but more commonly the information will only indicate different degrees of elevation of risk, as with the breast cancer susceptibility genes, *BRCA1* and BRCA2 (see Section 3.4). The degree to which interventions are possible to reduce or eliminate the health risk also varies greatly.

There are several ethical grounds of the practice of confidentiality of health information generally, and they have implications for how genetic information should be treated in family contexts. First, and perhaps most obviously, maintaining confidentiality typically prevents various possible harms to the patient, such as discrimination in employment or insurance. Second, since the information is obtained only with the patient's consent and cooperation, the patient should control who has access to it. Third, the information is about the patient and so the patient has the greatest interest in it and in who has access to it. Fourth, the medical profession in most countries promises to patients, either explicitly or implicitly, that their medical information will be treated confidentially.

In the case of genetic information with important consequences for family members' reproductive choices or health, it is generally only the second of these reasons that justifies maintaining confidentiality by not providing the information to affected family members without the patient's consent. Providing the information to family members will typically not harm the patient, the information is equally about the family member who consequently has a comparable interest in obtaining it, and confidentiality need not be promised to patients in these circumstances.

Patients can have in such circumstances a moral obligation to provide such information to potentially affected family members, and many believe that it should be permissible at least in some cases for health care providers to do so as well, without the consent of the patient, if necessary. In implementing genetic screening or testing programmes in developing countries, health ministries and professional organizations should consider incorporating this limit on confidentiality to reflect the special feature of genetic information, emphasizing that it is typically about families, not just individual patients. Because there may be special circumstances, either individual or cultural, that may warrant not giving information to affected family members in particular cases, for example if doing so will likely lead to harm or violence to the individual, an institutionalized process should be established to evaluate individual cases of breaches of patient confidentiality without the patient's consent in order to inform affected family members.

8.3.2 Discrimination and stigmatization

While there may be reason to limit confidentiality in cases of affected family members, because of the special nature of genetic information, its typically greater potential for discrimination and stigmatization provides reason to develop especially strong protection for genetic information in other contexts before genetic screening or testing programmes are initiated.

As genetic information about particular individuals, and sometimes groups as well, makes it possible to predict individuals' future health problems with varying degrees of probability, the information is potentially valuable to individuals for the prevention of disease, for therapy for the disease, or for planning their lives when neither prevention nor therapy are possible. However, this predictive power makes the information also valuable for others who may use it to wrongly discriminate against or stigmatize the individual in many social contexts. Employers may use the information to deny employment to individuals who may have potentially expensive future health problems. Health insurers may use the information in risk-rated health insurance to increase insurance rates substantially or to deny insurance altogether.

Many of these risks can be expected to increase in developing (and many developed) countries in the future. Responsibilities to provide health care are being shifted from the public sector to the private sector in many countries, where private insurers make use of risk rating for health insurance. As a wider range of genetic tests become available and their cost continues to decline, the incentives and abilities of insurers to use this information to discriminate against individuals with risks of developing serious disease will increase. Since genetic risks are viewed by many, even if often incorrectly, as impossible to reduce or eliminate, they may be given unduly great weight in these contexts.

The stigmatization of people carrying genes creating risks for serious disease can often have serious psychological consequences, not just social consequences with respect to labelling as diseased or unhealthy an individual who remains healthy and who has not yet developed, and may never develop, the disease in question. Being labelled as having "bad" genes can have a variety of serious social and psychological consequences for individuals, and this stigmatization may be stronger and more common where the levels of education and understanding of genetics is low.

Perhaps the most serious worry about genetic discrimination is in health insurance. WHO and many other international and national bodies concur that access to at least a basic level of health care is a human right and a requirement of equity or justice. Basic health care services should be available to all people and not just to those with the ability to pay for them. Since health care services are often expensive, with individuals' needs highly variable and unpredictable, they are difficult to budget for and so are typically provided through some form of insurance; usually social insurance within a national health system, but increasingly in many countries, at least in part, by private health insurance. If individuals are subject to risk rating for health insurance, and increasing amounts of information become available to insurers about genetic risks, many people will face large differences in their health insurance costs from genetic risks; they will be denied health insurance, or be unable to afford it at all. This will seriously undermine the universal provision of health care.

There is a compelling ethical case grounded in equity for community rating of either social or private health insurance in order to spread the costs of individuals' health risks across the larger community. Moreover, genetic risks are a paradigm of risks that are morally undeserved and which should not affect people's cost of or access to health care. Even if individuals may be responsible for some health risks due to their behavior, which is itself problematic, there is no plausible sense in which they are responsible for their genome and the health risks it generates, that is, for their good or bad luck in the "genetic lottery." Rating health insurance by health risks, whether based on genetic or other factors, has the intended, though from the standpoint of the social purpose of health insurance, perverse effect of making it more difficult, or even impossible, for individuals to obtain health insurance who may need it the most.

Genetic screening or testing should not be introduced in a country without first having clear and enforceable legislation prohibiting the use of genetic tests for health insurance or the use of genetic information by insurance companies in decisions to offer or deny health insurance, or in setting health insurance rates for individuals or groups. A similar ethical case can be made for not allowing use of genetic information in underwriting of disability insurance, at least for reasonable cover.

The ethical case against the use of genetic information in life insurance underwriting, however, is less clear. While individuals who learn that they have a serious genetic health risk should not be deprived of health insurance, they should not be able to amass large amounts of life insurance on the basis of serious health risks of which they, but not their life insurer, are aware. However, life insurance is not always used only for compensation in the case of death. For example, in some countries it is widely used as collateral for loans on a house, without which the rate of interest on the loan would rise substantially. In that context, denial of life insurance on the basis of genetic information results in unfair discrimination in access to housing.

Similar ethical concerns apply to the use of genetic testing by employers or potential employers. Current health problems that would prevent a person from carrying out the duties of employment, even when employers have made reasonable accommodations for illness or disabilities, can justifiably be used in employment decisions. But genetic conditions that constitute risks for future health problems should not be used to bar otherwise qualified people from employment. If and when they prevent the individual from continuing in employment, they can be dealt with appropriately. Nor should people be denied employment because their genetic condition creates a risk of high future health care costs to their employer when health insurance is provided through employment, since this is in effect to deny them both health insurance and employment on the basis of a genetic condition creating future health risks. As in the case of health insurance, countries should not introduce genetic screening or testing without first having clear and enforceable legal prohibitions of the use of genetic information in employment decisions.

In some countries there may be deeper concerns based on religious or other cultural views about the acceptability of genetic screening and testing, often because abortion is associated with the practices but sometimes even when it is not. Countries will make their own decisions about whether these practices are compatible with their particular culture, laws, religion, and traditions, and more generally about the limits they wish to impose on the use of new genetic knowledge and interventions. It is important that this deliberation and decision-making is as open, inclusive, and democratic as possible. Especially because the potential future health benefits from genomics are substantial, societies should attempt to accommodate reasonable differences among their members on these issues.

8.4   GENDER ISSUES

In societies in which there is deep-seated bias and discrimination against women, genetic information can be withheld or used in ways deeply prejudicial to them (Rothenberg and Thomson, 1994; Davis, 2001). In strongly patriarchal societies, common in many countries, it is especially important to ensure that women are not subject to coercive pressure from within the family or community to pursue or not to pursue genetic testing. Publicly funded awareness and counselling programmes should be established to support women in making decisions about genetic testing on the basis of their own needs and interests. In addition, the consent process should include means to try to identify and prevent any form of coercion. In some countries, similar problems regarding coercion for sex selection of the fetus have arisen which have often proved difficult to prevent (see below). This underscores the special importance of public responsibility for supporting and promoting women's rights in countries without strong traditions of respecting the reproductive freedom of women and with substantial gender inequalities. If this responsibility is not carried out, the introduction of genetic testing has the potential to reduce rather than enlarge women's reproductive freedom. As new options arise, they will not be able to make free and uncoerced choices.

Genetic information can also be used to discriminate or stigmatize in the context of other social practices. For example, in the case of arranged marriages families may seek genetic information about potential spouses of their children. This information can make women unmarriageable if they are known to have genes for serious diseases, or it can subject them to physical and other harms if they give birth to children with diseases for which they are deemed responsible. In countries or cultures with strong discriminatory practices against women, special measures will be needed to protect them against stigmatization or discrimination on the basis of genetic information. Governments and other organizations should undertake an assessment of the special risks to women (and ethnic or cultural groups) in their countries from potential disclosure of genetic information before genetic research, screening, or testing goes forward, so as to limit the harms to those taking part in these programmes.

In many developing countries, abortion services are either not widely available or are prohibited by law except in a very narrow range of circumstances. Post conception genetic testing is typically undertaken with the intent to abort the pregnancy if the fetus is found to have the condition for which it was tested. In the absence of any therapeutic options for the fetus or the child after birth, and where ending the pregnancy is typically either not possible, or possible only under illegal and unsafe conditions, it is problematic whether public resources should be devoted to post conception genetic testing programmes. Moreover, better educated women in such countries are often able to obtain abortion services, despite their illegality, either within their own country or abroad. Genetic testing programmes in such circumstances can be harmful to women who lack the means to act safely on the information obtained.

Genetic information can also be a means to carry out sex selection and thus prevent the birth of female babies. Non-therapeutic sex selection by amniocentesis using chromosomal analysis, or later in pregnancy using sonogram technology, to determine the sex of the fetus, has received public attention and governmental response in several countries. In India, the use of sex selection to avoid the birth of female babies has had a substantial effect on the sex ratio of the population in some areas of the country. The Indian case is instructive because it displays some of the features that can make selection of offspring for non-therapeutic reasons ethically problematic. First, being female is not what might be called a natural disadvantage (indeed, it is a biological advantage in terms of longevity), but is a disadvantage only in the context of substantial prejudice and discrimination against women. Likewise, being male is largely not a natural or biological advantage, but a social advantage only in the context of these unjust social practices. It is the prejudice and discriminatory practices that should be changed, rather than preventing the birth of female babies which can have the effect of reinforcing unjust discrimination against women. Second, a stable sex ratio is a public good which among other things affords members of a monogamic society a reasonable chance to marry; a society can justifiably intervene in even rational individual choices to select for certain traits when doing so is necessary to protect an important public good.

For these reasons, but mainly because it was perceived that sex selection reflects a societal bias against female children, the Indian Government has taken a variety of steps to prevent selection against and abortion of female fetuses, although legal prohibitions have not been strongly enough enforced to be effective. Professional associations could often do more to regulate their members in this regard and the World Medical Association should exert pressure on its member associations to put more effort into controlling individual physicians' conduct in participating in sex selection.

Recent advances in sperm-selection technology, or "semen sexing," allow the separation of X- and Y-bearing spermatozoa so that fertilization can yield either female or male offspring, respectively. As this procedure advances, sex selection before conception is becoming a realistic option at relatively low cost. Sex-linked diseases can then be prevented before an embryo is conceived and without aborting the embryo or fetus. However, sperm selection can also be used for sex selection that does not prevent disease, but only reflects various social prejudices against women.

Sex selection is a result of deep-seated, entrenched beliefs and values in societies that have long histories of subordinating and devaluing women, and long-term public education strategies will be needed to combat them effectively.

8.5   EUGENICS

The specific ethical issues discussed above, informed consent, confidentiality, and discrimination and stigmatization, are all coloured by broader concerns about eugenics (Paul, 1995). The very power of the genetics revolution for our understanding of the genetic bases of human nature and for prevention or treatment of disease also gives rise to serious concerns in many people. For along with the understanding of our genetic inheritance and the role genes play in determining phenotype may come the potential to control and change human nature. Moreover, the belief that the genetic pool or inheritance of the population could be improved is not new to the Human Genome Project and contemporary genomics. From the 1870s to the 1940s, eugenics movements existed in many countries, and culminated in the Nazi eugenics programme whose unprecedented evils permanently discredited eugenics and largely ended the eugenics movement.

Nevertheless, it is important to understand what the source of the immorality of these historical eugenics movements was in order to avoid their mistakes in the contemporary genomics era. The charge that a particular practice is eugenic is often used to end discussion of the practice without making clear either what is meant by calling the practice eugenic or what precisely makes it wrong. Yet the core concern of eugenicists for human betterment through selection is considered by many people not in itself immoral, although eugenicists' means of achieving it were often unethical. Of course these historical movements were complex and varied in many ways, but several key features that led to their deeply immoral outcomes can be identified, and must be avoided in contemporary genomics.

One important feature of eugenics movements was a concern with what they believed to be a degeneration of the gene pool, which they sought to reverse by encouraging the "fit" to increase their reproduction and discouraging the "unfit" from reproducing. But the fit and unfit were commonly determined by racial, class, and national prejudices and stereotypes that still persist today in much of the developed and developing world, and that must be avoided in our use of the powers of the new genetics.

A second feature was belief in the heritability of behavioural traits and a biological basis for social problems, and a biological remedy for them. Reproduction was thus seen as having social consequences and hence was a legitimate matter of social concern, which often led to coercive control of reproduction by the state in support of eugenic goals. Between 1900–1910 many thousands of women in countries such as Sweden and the United States were involuntarily sterilized or otherwise coerced in their reproductive choices. Some recent policies in a few developing countries have also had coercive eugenic components. With greater capacity to control reproductive choices and outcomes now, individuals', and in particular women's, right to reproductive freedom must be properly respected.

The eugenics movements also failed to recognize adequately the concept of value pluralism, that is individuals', cultures', and societies' very different conceptions of what constitutes a good person, way of life, and society. As a result, eugenicists tended to favour people like themselves and to be intolerant of different personal and social ideals. With greater control over heredity and the kinds of people there will be, tolerance of different values and ideals will be essential, while also publicly debating appropriate limits on genetic selection.

Some have seen statism, and an active role of the state in reproductive choices and policies, as one of the fundamental wrongs of the eugenics movements. Although state involvement certainly increased the magnitude of the moral wrongs and even horrors of many eugenic programmes, state involvement is not necessary to perpetrate eugenic wrongs, and such concerns cannot be fully alleviated by keeping the state out of reproductive choices and policies. People can suffer harm from the cumulative effects of uncoerced eugenic choices of individuals, for example in stigmatizing them with particular genetic conditions or leading to discrimination against them in employment or insurance. However, the concern about statism underscores the fact that reproduction always takes place in a social context of unequal political, economic or social power. This hierarchy of power will almost certainly impinge to some degree on practices to achieve eugenic ends. Critical questions about any such practices will therefore include who has the power to select, and who defines such key notions as "better," "defective," or "healthy." The case of sickle cell disease is a useful cautionary reminder that the so-called "bad" gene for this disease is in some circumstances beneficial in protecting its carriers against malaria.

Finally, at the heart of many ethical concerns with eugenics are issues of justice and the sacrifice of some individuals' interests for the sake of some greater social good. Many historical eugenics movements and programmes identified an "underclass" whose genes were not wanted and who, through involuntary sexual segregation, stigmatization and denigration, sterilization, and even murder, paid a heavy and unjust price. The inequalities of social and political power noted above to a great extent made these injustices possible. A major task for contemporary genomics is to ensure that the interests and rights of individuals are not unjustly sacrificed for the benefit of some greater social good.

Some have seen the difference between earlier eugenics movements and contemporary clinical genetics in the different perspectives of each. The eugenics perspective was social, a public health focus on the gene pool and the health and welfare of the population. By contrast, the focus of clinical genetics is typically individual, providing a service to meet the desires of individual parents. But the population perspective is not in itself ethically suspect; there seems nothing ethically wrong, for example, in programmes to eradicate smallpox or polio, or genes that cause serious disease, from the population. The question is rather whether the social goal is ethical and pursued in a just manner.

In seeking to reap the fruits of contemporary genomics the moral failings of the historical eugenics movements must be avoided: race, class, and national prejudices; failure, particularly through state coercion, to respect individuals' human rights to reproductive freedom; intolerance of different views of a "good person," life and society; and abuse of inequalities of power and unjustly sacrificing the rights and interests of individuals for a supposedly greater social good. However, practices should not be dismissed as ethically unacceptable simply on the basis of loose charges that they are eugenic. There is too little unambiguous meaning to that charge and it should be replaced with a clear account of what specific features make the practices wrong.

8.6   THE DISABILITY RIGHTS MOVEMENT'S CHALLENGE TO GENETIC SCREENING AND TESTING

A serious challenge to genetic screening and testing programmes has been raised by members of disability rights movements in many countries (Parens and Asch, 2000). They argue that these programmes do not share the traditional medical goal of preventing or treating disease in individuals, but instead seek to prevent the existence of people with disabilities. Prenatal screening or testing is typically done with the goal of identifying potential parents at risk of genetically passing on serious disease, or identifying an affected fetus so that the pregnancy can be terminated. This is criticized as eugenic, replacing "defective" with "non-defective" individuals, rather than providing therapy to benefit existing individuals. Of course, if replacement were to involve killing people, then there is no dispute that it would be deeply wrong, but here the goal is to ensure that healthy instead of unhealthy people will be born.

Why do many in the disability rights movement view this form of replacement as unethical? They have raised several points. First, the disadvantages of most impairments are due mainly to the failure of society to accommodate disabled persons. Second, typical views about the lives of disabled people are often based on prejudices, stereotypes, and other false beliefs, with the result that disabled people themselves rate their own quality of life higher than the non-disabled rate it. This is in part because people are often able to adjust to their disabilities through processes of adaptation: new learning and skills development that improve their functional performances; coping, adjusting expectations to reflect impaired abilities, thereby increasing satisfaction with their accomplishments; and accommodation, changing life plans to better fit their impaired abilities. Third, only a very few genetic disorders, such as Lesch-Nyhan or Tay-Sachs disease, are so severe as to make the lives of people who have them perhaps not worth living. The vast majority of conditions for which genetic testing is now and will, in the future, be possible are not so severe; they leave an affected individual with a life that from the individual's perspective is clearly worth living, a life valued by the person whose life it is. Fourth, disabled people have made many positive contributions to the lives of others and to society. Finally, some worry that genetic screening and testing are part of broader undesirable pressures towards normalization, conformity, and intolerance of difference.

How do defenders of genetic testing and screening respond to the disability rights movement's critique? First, although the social disadvantage of many impairments could and should be reduced by changing society to better accommodate people with disabilities, even after doing so there will often still be some residual disadvantage for people with serious conditions. This may be particularly true in countries where resources available to accommodate persons with disabilities are limited. Second, the process of adaptation is typically burdensome and costly for disabled people, and often only partially successful, again, particularly in countries where the availability of health care and rehabilitative services is severely limited. Third, even though some people with disabilities adjust sufficiently to give them as good or even better quality lives than non-disabled people, whether this will be so cannot be known for any individual at the time of genetic testing. So long as a particular disability is a disadvantage for the entire class of people with it, it is reasonable to try to prevent it. Fourth, the process of coping can be ethically problematic when it involves acceptance of a significantly limited life. Though a person may through coping remain satisfied with their life, the life itself may remain significantly limited and diminished; again, satisfaction with one's life as a result of severely limited prospects for improvement is not an adequate measure of how good the life is. Finally, to the extent that treating and accommodating disabilities imposes significant costs and burdens on caregivers as well as on society as a whole, society can reasonably seek to prevent disabilities in order to avoid those costs, particularly in developing countries where resources are often substantially limited. Each of the points made by disability advocates noted above is valid and important. Defenders of genetic testing argue that there remain, nevertheless, good reasons to attempt to prevent serious disabilities through genetic screening and testing.

Disabled people often make another argument against using genetic testing and screening to avoid the birth of disabled individuals. They see society's message in supporting genetic testing for the conditions they have as being that it would have been better if they had never been born, a message that they and others quite understandably reject. Supporters of genetic testing argue that seeking to ensure that children will be born as healthy as possible need not have this message and is not in conflict with recognizing the full and equal moral status of disabled people, including their right to health care and other services to meet their needs. In this view, the message of genetic testing is directed at the disadvantage or suffering that serious disease or disability can cause, not at persons with the disease or disability. The message is that it would be better if children were born healthy and without the disease; the message is directed at the disability, not at people who have the disability. The desirability of preventing serious genetically transmitted disabilities has no implications for how people with those disabilities can or should be treated, and, in particular, does not justify their mistreatment in any way.

The case for genetic testing and screening to prevent genetically transmitted disabilities may be even stronger in some developing countries, where they often carry greater stigma and can constitute more serious disadvantages because of more limited resources available to treat or accommodate them. The prevention of serious disease through genetic screening or testing appears to many to be a legitimate public health goal, just as the goal of reducing or eliminating serious communicable disease is not an unethical eugenic practice.

8.7 NONTHERAPEUTIC GENETIC INTERVENTIONS: GENETIC ENHANCEMENTS

Historical eugenics movements sought to improve the gene pool principally through encouraging selective breeding. In the modern genomics era the possibility will exist in the future, though how far in the future is unclear, for the exercise of some control over individuals' genetic inheritance not just to eliminate disease, but to enhance normal traits (Parens, 1998). Some have condemned any nontherapeutic use of genetics to select and control the genetic inheritance of children as eugenic and unethical; they support absolute bans on all such uses. Others have taken a more measured position that allows for the possibility of genetic enhancement, if done within specific ethical limits.

Some consider human reproductive cloning a form of nontherapeutic enhancement. It is a point of consensus, even among those who may otherwise disagree about whether human reproductive cloning could ever be ethically acceptable under any circumstances, that at the present time its risks are far too great to permit the practice to take place (see Section 8.8).

Genetics now provides little evidence of links between specific genes and important behavioural traits, but work in behavioural genetics does support a significant genetic as well as environmental contribution to many behavioural traits. While significant genetic enhancement is still a hypothetical possibility and by no means a near-term prospect, either in developed or developing countries, we address it briefly here because it has been a significant source of public concern about the potential for misuse of new genetic knowledge and powers. If at some point in the future it becomes possible safely to enhance, for example, individuals' memory, intelligence, or immune system, doing so would likely be beneficial to almost everyone in most social contexts. These traits are "all purpose means," useful in nearly any plan of life. Any enhancements of children undertaken by their parents should be of traits like these. Enhancements of specific traits should not be undertaken if they would substantially narrow a person's opportunity when an adult autonomously to choose his or her own way of life.

Some object to any possible use of genetic interventions to select for or to shape and enhance normal traits as "playing God" an improper practice of seeking to design one's children. However, it is hard to see why trying to select against and to intervene to prevent the genetic transmission of disease is not equally playing God, though most people do not object to it in principle. Moreover, parents in nearly all societies are considered to have a responsibility to use a variety of environmental means to help their children develop and enhance their capacities, and they typically have substantial, although not unlimited, discretion in how they raise and shape their children. For example, parents have a responsibility to have their children vaccinated against a variety of diseases; if it became possible instead to use genetic means to enhance their children's immune systems against disease it is hard to see why it would, in principle, be wrong to do so. Of course, sometimes the effect of vaccinations is only for a limited period of time, whereas germ-line genetic interventions would affect future generations as well as the individual. While germ- line interventions cannot be ruled out as always unethical, their greatly increased risks mean that they should not be undertaken until the technology involved is sufficiently developed to provide a clearly favourable risk-benefit ratio (see Section 8.8). In general, interventions to prevent or treat serious disease will have more favourable risk-benefit ratios than most enhancements of normal functions.

It would be a mistake to believe that genetic interventions would change a child's essential identity in some deep way, whereas environmental interventions only bring out a fixed identity that is already present. There is no fixed phenotype that environmental efforts merely bring out; rather a range of phenotypes are possible, according to the different environments that parents might provide. Likewise, particular genetic interventions would also develop the phenotype in a particular direction. It is the nature and goal of the intervention, not whether it is genetic or environmental, that determines its ethical acceptability.

There are a variety of reasons to restrict who could offer genetic enhancements to parents for their children. As noted in the section on eugenics (Section 8.5), concerns about power inequalities are ever present and if governments were to attempt to employ genetic enhancements the potential for abuse — such as enhancements that might have social benefits but not be of benefit to the individual — increases substantially. However, all enhancements of normal function by governments cannot be ruled out in advance as ethically unacceptable; for example, many governments now fluoridate their water supplies in order to enhance their citizens' capacity to resist tooth decay. This enhancement is not ethically problematic merely because it is undertaken by government rather than individuals.

Societies have a moral obligation grounded in equity or justice and human rights to ensure access to health care for their citizens. A fundamental part of the moral importance of health care is its role in maintaining normal function, and in turn helping to secure equality of opportunity for persons that serious disease and disability can undermine. Genetic enhancements of normal function, on the other hand, do not serve justice in this way and if and when they become possible, will almost certainly not be regarded as part of the social obligation to provide health care to all members of society. Instead, they will likely be both available on an ability-to-pay basis, and generally expensive.

This means that enhancements would be available to the rich and not to the poor — the rich would be able to confer on their children not just social advantages, as they do now, but genetic advantages as well. The result could be a substantial widening of inequalities between developed and developing countries, as well as of inequalities within societies between the well-off and the worse-off. Particularly in many developing countries, where there are often very great inequalities between a very small, very privileged minority and a very poor general citizenry, the potential for widening inequalities is substantial.

This is perhaps the greatest ethical concern about possible future capacities to use genetics to significantly enhance important normal human functions — the unfairness of further widening already unjust inequalities of opportunity and well being between the rich and the poor.

The non-therapeutic use of genetic technology for enhancement of normal function may not be inherently unethical, but it raises a number of ethical concerns that must be addressed if and when it becomes possible.

8.8   GENE THERAPY, STEM CELL THERAPY AND HUMAN CLONING

Current approaches to research in human gene- or stem cell therapy are outlined in Sections 3.9 and 3.10, and the problems of regulation of work of this kind are discussed in Section 6.7. These rapidly moving fields are raising a number of ethical issues. Although the issues arising from gene therapy have been widely debated, and there is a considerable degree of agreement about how they should be handled, the position regarding stem cell therapy and its relationship to human reproductive cloning is still in a state of flux.

The distinction between somatic-cell and germ-cell gene therapy is described in Section 3.9. Somatic-cell gene therapy does not raise any fundamentally new ethical issues because, in principle, it is little different to organ transplantation or other therapy. Thus work in this field is based on the ethical principles applied to any form of human experimentation or therapy. Germ-cell gene therapy is different in this respect, principally because it has the potential to alter the genetic make-up of future generations, which would have had no input into the decision-making involved. However, as discussed in Section 6.4, research into human germ-cell gene therapy is prohibited in most countries, mainly on the grounds that since so little is known about the dangers of this procedure, and because there have been so few successes in somatic-cell gene therapy to date, the risks are too great at the moment to allow research in this field to proceed. If and when somatic-cell gene therapy is developed to the stage at which it is both effective and safe, and if there are severe genetic diseases which could only be cured by germ-cell therapy, the ethical issues of this approach may have to be revisited. If extensive animal studies were to show that it is effective, it is difficult to see why it would raise major ethical issues if used to eradicate a lethal genetic disease from a family; some would not even rule out the possibility of germ-line enhancement in the future.

The ethical issues regarding human embryonic stem cell research directed at cell therapy are more controversial. As pointed out in Section 3.10, although a great deal of research is being directed towards obtaining stem cells for therapeutic purposes from different adult tissues, human embryonic stem cells are currently the only cell populations which have unequivocal potential for developing into the wide range of different adult tissues required for organ repair. Because of the potential of this field for treating a large number of intractable diseases of later life, it has been argued that there is a strong case for pursuing research directed at the properties of human embryonic stem cells. This raises important and complex ethical issues relating both to the moral status of human embryos and to the relationship of the different manipulations that might be used in this work to genuine human reproductive cloning.

The ethical status of human embryos has been widely debated and is controversial (Robertson, 2001). An important distinction revolves around whether objections to research on embryos rest on rights-based or symbolic grounds. Those who view the human pre-implantation embryo as a full person with rights hold that its intentional destruction is equivalent to murder. Although many religious groups and others follow this line it conflicts with other widely held philosophical and moral views which hold that status as a person requires further development, such as at least a nervous system capable of sentience or even self-consciousness. The first sign of the presence of a nervous system is observed at about 14 days of development with the appearance of what is called the primitive streak. Even if lacking rights, the symbolic status of the embryo as the early stage of human development may create ethical issues in how it is treated. Based on these distinctions between rights and a symbolic view of the embryo, some countries, the United Kingdom, for example, have permitted research for specified purposes on embryos of less than 14 days development. Other countries have placed different limits on research on human embryos or banned it completely.

A second set of complex ethical issues in stem cell research arise from the practical problems of its application for organ therapy. As pointed out in Section 3.10, while methods may well be worked out to direct human embryonic stem cells to differentiate into particular cell or tissue types for transplantation and therapeutic effects, since these cells will not be derived from the patient they may well be rejected by the patient's immune system. In this case, one strategy might be to use the patient's nuclear DNA to create an embryo from which embryonic stem cells compatible with the patient could be derived. This would necessitate the transfer of nuclei from the patient's cells into an anucleated egg which would then be activated so that it grew to an early embryonic (blastocyst) stage. This is, in effect, an early step in human cloning, though, of course, it does *not* amount to true reproductive cloning unless there is the intention of introducing the embryo into a uterus.

This type of research raises a number of ethical issues. First, it would be necessary to create or otherwise obtain large numbers of human embryos which would be destroyed in the process of becoming recipient cells for the nucleus of patients who were to be treated. This would certainly raise ethical problems for those who believe that human embryos should not be destroyed. Even those who accord human embryos some symbolic status often accept the use of embryos "left over" from in vitro fertilization procedures and that would never be implanted. More controversial still is the creation of embryos solely with the intention of destroying them in order to produce cells to be used for activating adult nuclei. Undoubtedly other ethical issues will arise if this field continues to develop. The major problem will be how to obtain sufficient eggs required if therapeutic cloning becomes of widespread clinical value. Certainly this will exceed the numbers that are generated as part of in vitro fertilization. Would it be ethically acceptable to ask, or even pay, unrelated women to undergo repeated cycles of hormone treatment and egg retrieval for therapeutic uses? Would it be acceptable to obtain human eggs from cadavers or aborted fetuses? Even more controversially, would it be acceptable to use bovine eggs in which to develop human nuclei?

Those who do not view early embryos as having inherent moral status that forecloses their destruction may find no significant ethical barrier to obtaining human embryonic stem cells from early pre-implantation embryos for their use in research or therapy. Provided the distinction is maintained between therapeutic and reproductive cloning it may be reasonable to continue to explore different possibilities for generating sufficient eggs necessary for the therapeutic applications of this field. But if embryonic stem cell replacement therapy becomes safe and effective, there will be ethical issues related not just to the supply of eggs, but also to access to treatment for those who would benefit from these potentially revolutionary but extremely expensive forms of therapy.

A second ethical concern is that stem cell therapy, if it were perfected, might lead to genuine reproductive cloning by the replacement of an anucleate egg containing an adult nucleus in the uterus. But there seems little reason to believe that it is necessary to forgo the great potential benefits of therapeutic cloning in order to prevent human reproductive cloning. A much more reasonable position, reflected in both the Council of Europe's Convention on Human Rights and Biomedicine and

UNESCO's Universal Declaration on the Human Genome and Human Rights, is that the line between therapeutic cloning and reproductive cloning is quite clear and that reproductive cloning can be prohibited without impeding cloning for therapeutic purposes. It is unfortunate that the term "therapeutic" cloning has been used to describe work in this field (Vogelstein et al., 2002). While it will undoubtedly generate technology which could be misused for human reproductive cloning the distinction between the two is absolutely clear and would provide no problems for appropriate legislation.

Currently, there is a near universal consensus of opinion that the risks inherent in any attempt at human reproductive cloning at the present time would make doing so clearly unethical. Many also believe that human reproductive cloning would be unethical under any circumstances and that there is no ethical or medical basis for pursuing work on it. This view has been stated by WHO, and many countries have made it illegal to pursue work directed towards this end, or are in the process of doing so.

8.9   SUMMARY

The ethical issues arising from the applications of genome research are extremely complex and constantly changing. But although they present particular problems for different societies depending on their religious beliefs, social structure and cultural practices, they can be based on broad principles which are relevant to every society. Hence there is a major requirement for international leadership in developing a broad framework on which individual countries can develop their own codes of ethical practice as this field evolves in the future.

9. EDUCATION AND PUBLIC POLICY

Contents

9.1   INTRODUCTION

One of the major concerns voiced during the consultations which preceded this Report was the widespread lack of public awareness about the principles of genetics. This is a particularly serious problem because genetics will impinge on so many aspects of medical research and practice in the future. For example, genetic screening and testing, whether as part of research programmes in genetic epidemiology or for detecting carrier states for common genetic disease, requires that those who are screened have some basic understanding of genetic mechanisms. Although the explanation of the role of genetics in particular diseases is usually the responsibility of genetic counsellors, adequate counselling in a population in which there is very limited comprehension of genetics is extremely difficult to achieve.

This problem is compounded by the fact that lack of understanding of the fundamentals of genetics permeates throughout society, including the media, policy- makers, and even the medical profession itself. Hence, if it is to be prepared for a new variety of medical research and practice which relies heavily on genetic principles, it is vital that future planning for health care includes education in this field. Furthermore, unless this problem is tackled quickly, it will be very difficult for the developing countries to establish the structures in bioethics which are essential for any society which is pursuing medical research, particularly in genomics.

9.2   LEVEL OF KNOWLEDGE ABOUT GENETICS

From what little is known about the level of knowledge about genetics among different populations, it is clear that there is widespread misunderstanding of the mechanisms of inheritance. For example, in its report on Genetic Screening, the United Kingdom Nuffield Council on Bioethics (1993) examined the evidence available and came to the conclusion that there is widespread confusion, in particular about the nature of recessive genes and the meaning of carrier status. It encountered equal lack of knowledge of how genetic diseases are transmitted, which was often confused with notions about the inheritance of physical characteristics, such as height, eye colour, etc. It found that genetics is often mistaken for eugenics and that there are widespread concerns about stigmatization, which may or may not have a basis in fact.

Unfortunately, this lack of understanding of genetics also affects the work of some of the media and a great deal of misinformation is disseminated, leading either to public concern or to an exaggerated perception of the immediate benefits of genetic research. It extends to policy-makers and, particularly because of the paucity of politicians with scientific backgrounds, the quality of debate in many governments on genetics matters can be extremely poor. There are undoubtedly deficiencies in knowledge about genetics among many physicians; the introduction of genetics as part of the preclinical or clinical courses in medical schools is only a recent development and, because the field is moving so rapidly, many doctors are, or become, ill-prepared to assess the importance or relevance of genetic factors in disease.

Although in some countries specialist genetic centres and services have been developed, in many cases they are still inadequate in meeting the needs of the community, particularly in public education. Despite the fact that genetics now permeates every branch of medicine, as discussed earlier, its value to other specialities is not as yet fully appreciated.

It is clear that the situation in developing countries is even worse. In countries where general education and an informed media are lacking, the people are likely to be even less well-informed about genetics. Where no genetic services have been developed there will be few or no physicians or other health professionals who have had any training in delivering clinical genetics services or genetic counselling, let alone public education.

If there is to be a new era of medical practice in which genetics plays an important role, it is absolutely vital that these problems are solved before communities are exposed to medical research involving genetic screening and testing, let alone the applications of genetic intervention for the prevention or management of disease. One example will suffice to emphasize how things can go wrong if an education programme of this type is not put in place before a genetic screening policy is unleashed.

In the USA in the 1960s, sickle-cell anaemia was rediscovered as an important health problem and it was decided that there should be a blanket screen for the sickling disorders in some states. However, this was not combined with an adequate education programme about the nature of the disease and was not supported by any provisions for genetic counselling. In several states, laws were passed which made screening mandatory, again without any attempt at education. The result was large-scale public anxiety, stigmatization, job and health insurance discrimination, and many other undesirable effects; virtually nothing was achieved. This outcome has to be compared with the success of genetic screening programmes in Montreal, Canada and Sardinia, Italy which, because they were preceded by wide-scale public education programmes, turned out to be extremely successful (Scriver et al., 1984; Cao and Rosatelli, 1993).

In short, it would be extremely unwise for any form of "genetic medicine" to be introduced into countries in which there is a low level of knowledge about genetics among the public and where no genetic services or counselling facilities exist.

9.3   PUBLIC PERCEPTIONS OF BIOTECHNOLOGY AND GENETIC ENGINEERING

Because the potential medical applications of genomics will reflect a completely new approach to patient care, and knowing that the level of knowledge about the principles of genetics among the public is limited, it is important for the further development of this field that information is obtained about how it is viewed by different communities. Over the last 10 years several surveys have been carried to obtain information of this kind (Richmond et al., 1999). Most of them have attempted to learn more about how the public perceive such activities as biotechnology, genetic engineering, gene therapy, genetic testing, and related research. Under the sponsorship of the European Commission, surveys of the European public were performed in 1991, 1993 and 1996, and similar surveys were carried out in 1996 in Canada and in 1997 in New Zealand and Japan using the same approaches.

The results of these surveys showed a remarkable diversity of response among different populations. For example, in the 1997 survey only one third of Japanese had heard about the use of biotechnology to produce new medicines and vaccines, compared to two thirds of New

Zealanders. Approximately 50% of Europeans were familiar with the term biotechnology, ranging from 30% in Greece to 70% in Finland and Austria.

Looking at the trends over time there appears to be both an increase in knowledge but, at the same time, an increase in concern about these activities. For example, in 1991, surveys in Japan and New Zealand indicated that 76% of Japanese and 57% of New Zealanders thought that genetic engineering would be worthwhile for their country, while 20% and 8%, respectively, were worried about it. Yet in 1997, only 54% of Japanese and 32% of New Zealanders thought that genetic engineering would result in improvements in health; 12% of Japanese and 39% of New Zealanders thought that it might "make life worse" (Macer et al., 1997). In every country risk appeared to be related to perceived usefulness. After the 1996 surveys it was apparent that usefulness is a precondition of support for work of this kind; people are prepared to accept some risk as long as there is a perception of usefulness and no moral concern, and, importantly, moral issues seem to negate people's views on both use and risk.

The only country which has had a national vote on the future of the use of genetic engineering is Switzerland. In 1998, the Swiss voted by a 2:1 majority against a referendum to ban genetic engineering. Arguments supporting the ban were based on perceived risk for both human health and the environment together with ethical concerns, while those who opposed it focused on the deleterious effect it would have on medical research and on the development of therapeutic agents by the pharmaceutical industry. In particular, it was believed that it would lead to isolation of Switzerland from the mainstream of science. Opinion polls during the period running up to the vote showed a distinct change, with a considerable reduction in the number who opposed genetic engineering.

In 1998 a nationwide survey in the United States, commissioned by the National Center for Genome Resources, polled 1039 households across the country. The returns showed a wide range of understanding of the fields of biotechnology and genetics. For example, although 91% thought they understood the meaning of "gene" and 93% the meaning of genetic testing, less than 50% understood the meaning of the term human gene therapy. About 50% were aware that genetic tests were available, while 25% were not sure and 20% did not think they were available. While there was widespread uncertainty about the meaning of gene therapy and whether it had ever been successful, there was a surprisingly high level of acceptance of the technologies of genetic engineering: 93% for early diagnosis of disease; 86% for identifying people likely to develop a disease; 88% for determining whether an individual is a carrier. A surprising outcome of this survey was that public approval of genetic testing did not appear to relate to whether a disease could be treated. For example, 94% thought that patients should be advised by their physicians to be tested for the likelihood of developing a treatable cancer, yet 76% thought the testing should be extended to untreatable cancers. Interestingly, 22% of the public thought it was wrong to change the genetic make-up of human cells, regardless of the purpose, although this was a marked decrease from the 42% offering the same opinion 10 years earlier.

These examples of the studies reviewed by Richmond et al. (1999) are of importance for several reasons. First, they provide some indication of the public perception and feeling about developments in genomics and biotechnology. The level of response in some of these studies was remarkably high, indicating that there is considerable public interest in this field. This suggests that carrying out surveys of this kind may play an increasingly useful role in encouraging public debate on how far society should move in research and development relating to genomics while, at the same time, providing stimulation for the public to become better educated in the complex issues involved. Carried out sequentially, they also offer a very useful barometer of the public's perceptions of the ethical and moral problems presented by genomics, and hence provide governments and others with a yardstick for developing regulatory programmes. So far this approach has not been used widely in developing countries (see Section 7) but where it has the pattern of answers has been quite different to those of the developed countries (Richmond et al., 1999) (Box 9.1), bearing in mind that the studies are not broadly comparable due to different methodologies and the different questions asked.

As part of exercises of this type directed at trying to understand the public's perception of the biomedical sciences, it is important to include analyses of their concepts of science in general and not simply restrict reviews to areas specific to genomics (Office of Science and Technology, 2000). An analysis of public perspectives on human cloning and related areas of biomedical research, carried out by the Wellcome Trust in the United Kingdom, offers valuable guidelines to methods for developing programmes to test public reactions to scientific developments and also describes some of the pitfalls that may be encountered in this important work (Wellcome Trust, 1998).

Box 9.1   SURVEY ON PUBLIC AWARENESS, PERCEPTION AND ATTITUDE TOWARD
CLONING IN BANGKOK, THAILAND

The objective of this study was to investigate the status of awareness, perception, and acceptance of "cloning " technology among the Thai public residing in Bangkok in 2001. More than 2,500 people in 33 districts were interviewed, according to the sample size calculated by simple random sampling methodology. Results were classified and analysed with regard to sex, religion, age, educational background, and occupation. Members of the target group were those who had lived in Bangkok for 3 months or longer. The study was carried out during October to December 2001.

The study found that most of those surveyed were aware of the term "cloning." It was evident that the key contributing factor to this awareness was the availability of information from the media. However, more than one-third of this informed group showed some misunderstanding or confused perception of the technology's definition, probably due to inaccuracy of the information.

The majority of those surveyed felt that both cloning of humans and animals were beneficial and should be allowed, but animal cloning was more accepted than human cloning. The reasons for the difference of opinion regarding animal and human cloning may be attributed to lack of urgent necessity, ethical dilemmas, and potential negative effects.

Furthermore, this study also reported a correlation between perception of cloning technology and personal background of those surveyed. It was found that correct understanding of the definition of the technology, together with acceptance, decreased with age. Also, people with higher educational backgrounds, especially those at graduate school level, had a tendency to be more positive towards cloning. Differences in perception of the technology were shown to lead to differences in attitude. On the other hand, gender seemed to have no correlation with either perception or attitude toward the technology.

Source: Nares Damrongchai and Numkang Chaiput, National Center for Genetic Engineering and Biotechnology (BIOTEC). Corresponding author: E-mail: nares@biotec.or.th

Clearly, the monitoring of public perceptions of different aspects of genomic research, particularly as it relates to medical practice, will be of particular importance in the future, and should be encouraged by WHO for its Member States.

9.4   LACK OF ORGANIZATIONS FOR SETTING PUBLIC POLICY AND ETHICAL STANDARDS FOR GENOMICS

In Section 6, the lack of structures for the regulation of recombinant DNA technology in many countries was emphasized. During the consultations which preceded this Report it became clear that the same deficiencies exist in determining public policy and ethical standards, right across the field of human genetics and genomics. Furthermore, the correction of this situation was given a very high priority by many of those consulted.

Over recent years there has been an enormous amount of activity in many of the developed countries and on the part of a wide variety of international agencies in the field of bioethics as it relates to human genetics and its potential medical applications.

Although the precise mechanisms vary in detail, the general principles for developing public policy and ethical frameworks for the use of recombinant DNA technology have evolved along similar lines in many of the developed countries. In the United Kingdom, for example, it was decided that it would be valuable to have a bioethics council which was completely independent of government, the medical establishment, and research funding bodies. In 1992, the Nuffield Council on Bioethics was established, with a membership which included scientists with a knowledge of genetics, but also lawyers, theologians, industrialists, philosophers, and members of the general public of wide-ranging backgrounds. The Council anticipated developments in genetics and established a number of expert working parties to advise them on the ethical issues involved. Although it had no standing in law it rapidly gained the respect of government and provided a central, independent role in developing policy on ethical issues. At the same time, and as each new development appeared on the horizon, the government set up expert committees to report and advise on these issues, and with the advice from the Nuffield Council on Bioethics and similar bodies, appropriate legislation was developed. The principles for maintaining ethical standards in the field were made widely available to the universities and teaching hospitals, each of which have their own institutional bioethics committees for regulating medical research.

Most countries have followed a similar pattern of development, although in some the central advisory bodies are government-based and hence not entirely independent. Almost every country has a system of institutional ethical committees in place. Most large pharmaceutical companies also have their own ethics boards.

There are several examples of bioethics programmes in developed countries which are addressing issues of direct relevance to developing countries, and are working to facilitate capacity-building activities in these developing countries. The Canadian Programme on Genomics and Global Health at the University of Toronto, Toronto, Canada provides one case in point.

These national activities have been backed up by several international bodies that have developed bioethics programmes. In Europe, the two main institutions active in this field are the Council of Europe and the

European Commission. The Council of Europe's activities, which go back to the late 1970s, have included the recent drafting of a convention for the protection of human rights and dignity. The European Commission has dedicated funds for the promotion of collaborative research into bioethics through its Framework programmes, and has established a number of committees to examine particular ethical aspects of research, including those involving human embryos and reproduction and the ethical, legal and social aspects of the human genome. It has also established the Group of Advisors on the Ethical Implications of Biotechnology, which was reconstituted in 1997 under the title European Group on Ethics in Science and New Technologies.

The Human Genome Organization is, through its Ethics Committee, also playing an important role in defining the ethical issues of the genome project and UNESCO has a number of major ongoing activities in bioethics. Over the last two years, WHO has been developing strategic priorities for a programme of work in the ELSI (ethical, legal and social implications) of genomics. In 2001, it announced a major new Ethics in Health initiative through which its current and future activities in bioethics will be focused. Several international public-interest organizations have worked on bioethics, including the Rural Advancement Foundation International, and the Council for Responsible Genetics.

This extraordinary expansion of bodies which are setting guidelines for the ethical issues arising from advances in genomics, while it underlines the widespread concern about developments in this field, poses a number of difficulties. First, because many of these organizations have a regional basis, their perspective of particular ethical issues may not always be germane to those of other countries, particularly those of the developing world. As discussed in Section 8, although some of these issues are all encompassing, many need to be examined in the light of the different social, religious and cultural backgrounds of particular populations.

Second, there is no single body which can move quickly and provide advice to governments on particularly sensitive issues. The result is that some controversial aspects of genetic manipulation may be acceptable in some countries and not in others at any one time. Finally, it is difficult for countries which have not yet developed any ethical framework for human genetics or recombinant DNA technology to know exactly where to turn for appropriate advice.

In the field of genomics what was thought to be impossible today is often commonplace tomorrow. It is vital therefore that one central body, and this could be WHO, takes the lead in trying to amalgamate the work of all these institutions and establishes a mechanism whereby new ethical issues can be rapidly debated and a consensus of advice made available to governments, and which, at the same time, will act as a focal point for providing advice to countries in which recombinant DNA technology is in the early stage of development.

9.5 REQUIREMENTS FOR EDUCATION AND POLICY-MAKING IN THE GENOMICS ERA

9.5.1 Public education

The requirements for public education in genetics will vary from country to country. While in many developed countries some genetics has been introduced into high school curricula there are still many deficiencies, particularly relating to tensions between whose responsibility it is to place this teaching in an ethical framework and how this should be done. In many of the developing countries in which facilities for education are limited it is vital that some form of instruction is incorporated as education programmes evolve. There is a major opportunity for forming networks of programmes for education of teachers in this field, both in the developed and developing countries. Currently, the International Union of Biological Sciences has a programme directed at bioethics teaching in schools.

Since raising the level of genetics teaching in schools will be a slow process, it is vital that major efforts are made to increase public awareness of developments in genetics through adult education. Experiences in trying to educate the population about the high frequency of a single genetic disease in Cyprus and Sardinia suggest that the best approach is through the media, particularly television. For this to be successful there needs to be a well-informed body of science journalists and, here again, there are major opportunities for regional networking. Some good models already exist for this purpose. For example, in the United Kingdom both government and charitable bodies have developed networks between scientists and the media such that the press and television industry can obtain expert advice as new scientific developments occur. Many research institutions run open days for the media and a variety of organizations are involved in furthering public understanding, awareness and appreciation of science. These approaches constitute an ideal way forward for developing regional networks for public education in the developing countries. Advocacy on the part of WHO could do much to encourage this activity.

9.5.2   Health care professionals

It is becoming increasingly important that genetics becomes an integral part of the training of physicians, nurses and other health care professionals. Surveys carried out over recent years suggest that even in some of the developed countries there are still major deficiencies and that teaching of the ethical framework that should underlie genetic medicine is often limited. Because the field is moving so quickly it is equally important that there are provisions for postgraduate education in this field in every speciality. It is important that WHO passes on this message to the governments of its Member States.

9.5.3   The educational role of clinical genetics services

As discussed in detail in Section 5, it is important that countries establish a strategy for the development of clinical genetics. Centres for this purpose can be either attached to university teaching hospitals or run as part of government health services. They require physicians who have been trained in clinical genetics, supported by technical staff and, in particular, nurses or related health professionals who have been trained in genetic counselling. Even in developed countries, governments have been slow to appreciate the importance of this field, and clinical genetics has remained low on the list of health care priorities. In the case of the developing countries this must be a high priority for the post-genomic period of research and health care development. Without adequate counsellors the introduction of any form of genetic screening and testing into populations will be fraught with difficulties, as described earlier in this section (see Section 9.2).

The importance of moving quickly towards the development of genetic services of this type cannot be overemphasized. As well as providing clinical and counselling expertise, such services will have the effect of generating a critical mass of individuals with the background and training required to develop national structures for the regulation of genetic research, establishing ethical standards (as outlined in Section 8), and developing programmes of public education in genetics.

The provision of sufficient physicians and ancillary staff trained in medical genetics will be a considerable challenge and an important opportunity for both developed-developing country collaborations and the development of local and regional networking. WHO could provide invaluable support for these developments to Member States which request it.

9.6 SUMMARY

The applications of genomics for improving health raise a wide range of new organizational and ethical issues, all of which require a knowledge of the principles of genetics on the part of the public, media, medical profession, and health care policy- makers and governments. Genomics has the potential to make an important impact on health care for the future and it is vital therefore that society is prepared for the many new concepts that it will bring with it. This will only be achieved by improving the standard of education about the basics of genetics at every level, ranging from primary schools to adult populations. Because of the time-scale that will be required to achieve this end, and because of the speed of development and discovery in genomics, it is important that this process is started without delay.

10. Recommendations for WHO and Its Member States

Contents
10.1 Introduction
10.2 Recommendations
10.3 Closing summary and key messages

10.1 Introduction

Predictions about the advances for health care that will result from the further exploration of the human and pathogen genomes in the functional genomics phase of research are uncertain and constantly changing. In this rapidly moving scene, even the governments of those countries in which research in this field is well advanced are receiving conflicting advice about the relevant importance of genomics in planning health care for the future. While the ultimate benefits may be enormous, it is impossible to predict when they will become available for clinical practice and, in particular, which of them will be of greatest importance in improving the health of developing countries.

Throughout this Report we have seen that enough is known already to suggest that work in the post-genomic period will begin to make a major impact on clinical care, albeit slowly. However, the central message is that, because of the uncertainties about both the extent of these benefits for medical practice and the time-scale involved, it is vital to maintain a balance in medical research between genomics and more traditional and well-tried approaches of clinical practice, public health and clinical and epidemiological research. Indeed, it must be emphasized that genomic research will only yield its full potential if it is integrated alongside these disciplines.

A key concern is that the majority of the developing countries do not at present possess either the technological capacity or skill base to reap the potential benefits of genomics research and apply them to their health care needs. Furthermore, many countries have yet to establish the regulatory, ethical and policy frameworks that are required to address the economic, legal and social implications of this field, and safeguard against the potential risks and hazards of these technologies in the best interests of their populations.

The recommendations that follow are set in the context of the key issues that Member States will need to consider in planning for this new era, as have been described in this Report. It must be stressed that all WHO Member States will need to make their own assessments of this field and develop their future strategies in light of their particular priorities for health care, and in their own unique social and economic contexts. As outlined in these recommendations, countries will often benefit from working in partnership to address these concerns, both at a regional level, through collaborations between the developing countries and between developed and developing countries.

In furthering its objective of the attainment by all peoples of the highest possible level of health, and as a United Nations agency committed to the promotion of fundamental human rights, WHO has a key role to play in assisting its members states in realizing the potential of genomics to improve health care, while ensuring that the implications and risks of these technologies are addressed adequately. Overall, it must work in support of its Member States to ensure that genomics is used to reduce, rather than to exacerbate, existing inequalities in global health. These recommendations describe how WHO could further this goal through enhancing its ability to respond to requests for technical cooperation from Member States, exercising its normative function to set overarching principles and harmonize standards for the genomics era, and adopting a strong advocacy position on a number of critical issues.

10.2   RECOMMENDATIONS

10.2.1   Technical Cooperation Between WHO and its Member States

1.   Assessing the health impacts of genomics research to support informed priority setting

Genomics research is progressing at a remarkable speed and the coming decades are likely to see an enormous expansion of this field, with important potential for clinical application to benefit health care globally. At present, there is widespread uncertainty among governments and their health advisors in countries in which genomics research is well-established about the way in which health care will develop in the postgenome period, and the position is likely to be even more confusing for many governments of the developing world. In order to support an informed priority-setting process in research and health care planning, all Member States will need access to accurate information on advances in genomics research and their potential for health care application in comparison with existing practice.

To support its Member States, WHO should develop the capability to examine critically advances in genomics for their potential for health care, and disseminate this information to governments in a timely manner. In particular, WHO should develop the mechanisms required to evaluate such advances in comparison with more conventional approaches to medical research and development, especially with regard to their likely cost-effectiveness and value to particular populations and environments within Member States. Such a function might require both the development of in-house expertise and the establishment of a panel of expert advisors from a wide spectrum of disciplines. Through these mechanisms, WHO could produce rapid, accessible and state-of-the-art reports to help governments plan their medical research and health care policies.

In practice, an approach similar to that outlined in Section 5 for assessing the value of genomics for the developing countries could be taken: providing advice to governments on those areas of genomics that are ready for immediate application for important health problems in their countries, giving them early warning of the outcomes of genomics research which are so advanced as to be extremely likely to be applicable in the near future, and disseminating accurate information on the progress of genomics research with more long-term prospects for application. Structured advice of this type would provide a more logical framework for setting priorities for research and development in health care in Member States.

2. Developing clinical genetics services and DNA technologies for other research fields

The development of clinical genetic services, based on easily transferable and well-tried clinical applications of DNA technology could provide immediate benefits to health care in many developing Member States, enabling the control of the common inherited disorders of haemoglobin, for example. In many cases, this approach will also be the simplest means of introducing DNA technology directly into clinical practice. Furthermore, it could enable the development of other crucial research fields, such as the genetic epidemiology of communicable and non-communicable diseases, which utilize very similar technologies. By establishing this technology in specialized clinical genetics centres, it can be easily transferred into other areas of medical research and care as it becomes relevant.

In order to establish clinical genetic services, Member States will need to develop sufficient numbers of clinicians trained in this field, backed up by technical staff and well-trained counsellors. Two main approaches are suggested which Member States could explore. First, many successful training programmes for technology transfer of this type have already been established by developed-developing country collaboration, a particularly valuable approach for countries in which there are no services of this type currently available. Second, and equally importantly, there are countries in most WHO regions in which services of this type have already been developed, and hence there are important opportunities for the development of local networking for training in this field.

Educational programmes to raise awareness of genetics among the public are a further essential prerequisite for the introduction of genetic services in Member States. Indeed, as discussed in Section 9, the introduction of clinical genetics also provides a valuable focus for raising the level of professional and public awareness of genetics and its implications.

WHO could play a major role in providing technical assistance to Member States to aid them in establishing centres for clinical genetics and genetic research programmes targeted to their particular health problems, through supporting regional meetings, the establishment of collaborative training programmes between developed and developing countries, and the development of local networking. Developing this capability may require a considerable expansion of existing WHO activities in human genetics, and the strengthening of in-house expertise in both clinical and community genetics. WHO has, however, already undertaken a great deal of preparatory work in this field and hence could move quickly in assisting its Member States in this regard.

3. Capacity building for genomics research and biotechnology in developing countries

A key conclusion of this Report is that it is vital that Member States in the developing world begin to develop appropriate technological capacities to make best use of the potential of genomics for their own health needs. For many such countries, an important priority will be to utilize the potential of pathogen and human genomics to develop new approaches for the control and management of communicable diseases. Although there are now major international research programmes addressing HIV/AIDS, malaria and tuberculosis, many of the important infections which are more localized in their occurrence will not attract funding from the global pharmaceutical industry due to the lack of market incentive. Responsibility for utilizing the potential of genomics to combat these diseases will undoubtedly fall largely to the individual countries and regions of the developing world.

Universities, public research institutions and the commercial sector all have crucial roles to play in research and development programmes focused on local health priorities. While biotechnology capacity is already well advanced in some of the developing countries, in others it is almost non-existent, and even where it is being developed there are major problems in retaining talented staff. Unless this imbalance between countries in terms of technological capacity in both academic and commercial settings is addressed, there is little chance that the potential of genomics to combat neglected diseases of the world's poor will be realized and existing inequalities in health care will be exacerbated still further as a result.

As a first step in developing strategic priorities for capacity building, Member States should consider undertaking analyses of their existing biotechnology capacity, both individually and at a regional level.

There are then several potential approaches to capacity building which Member States could explore. First, partnerships between academia, public research institutions and companies in developed and developing countries, and between the developing countries themselves, through the establishment of joint appointments for their scientists could be fostered to support the transfer of technologies and skills. Second, the continued development of local networking in those regions where there is evolving expertise in biotechnology will also be crucially important.

The concept of industrial partnerships between developed and developing countries, and among developing countries themselves, might constitute a particularly promising approach for Member States to advance. Pathogen genome screening and genomics for the purpose of identifying potential vaccine or therapeutic candidates is a long, complex and expensive process. Even if sufficient commercial incentives could be developed to encourage investment in neglected diseases, many large pharmaceutical companies do not have the capacity to deal with many of the infections which occur in localized parts of the world. On the other hand, the development of partnerships with an evolving biotechnology industry in the developing world, particularly if encouraged by tax or other government incentives, might be a much more attractive proposition.

By utilizing its convening power, WHO could play an important role in fostering the development of innovative partnerships between governments, academic and public sector research institutions, industry and other research funders aimed at fostering capacity building in biotechnology in Member States in the developing world. It could also respond to requests from individual Member States for technical assistance in capacity building in this research field as is considered appropriate.

4.   Capacity building for bioinformatics

Participation in genomics research requires the associated development of bioinformatics to store, analyse and interpret the vast quantities of data that are generated. Much of the data that in being produced from the genome sequencing projects and downstream functional genomics studies at genomics research institutions worldwide are being released freely into the public domain, and a number of sophisticated algorithms and other software resources are likewise available via the Internet without restriction. The establishment of adequate infrastructures and a critical mass of expertise for bioinformatics will be essential if Member States are to utilize this information for research towards their own health priorities.

As is the case with biotechnology, some developing countries have started to develop programmes for capacity building in bioinformatics, but many have yet to begin. There is already a critical shortage of manpower in this crucially important discipline, even in developed countries. Here too, Member States should consider undertaking assessments of their existing technological capacity and skill bases to identify existing shortfalls and provide a basis upon which to develop their strategic priorities for the future.

WHO could provide technical assistance to Member States in developing their bioinformatics capabilities through fostering regional networking, developed-developing country partnerships and short-term training programmes, with the specific objective of training young graduates in bioinformatics. The TDR Programme in WHO has already initiated training programmes in bioinformatics which could provide a starting point for further WHO involvement in this field.

5. Facilitating the development of ethical review structures and bioethics capacity

Individual Member States will need to develop detailed ethical frameworks to guide the conduct of genomics research and its medical application in their own unique social, cultural, economic and religious context.

As described below, this process must be guided by fundamental principles that have been agreed internationally. Currently, a major concern is that many countries which have either had no experience to date of recombinant DNA technology, or in which work of this kind is just starting, do not have the national or institutional ethical committee frameworks on which adequate regulatory programmes can be developed. Furthermore, in many Member States, there is a critical shortage of individuals trained in bioethics who can contribute to the analysis of the ethical issues raised by these technologies. Once again, Member States should consider exploring collaborative approaches between developed and developing countries, and between developing countries, to foster capacity building in this field.

WHO could play an important role in working with Member States to assist them in establishing appropriate ethical frameworks and disseminating the major principles upon which programmes of bioethics suited to local needs should evolve. It could also play a major role in supporting international and regional training programmes in bioethics.

10.2.2   WHO's Normative Function

6.   International leadership in establishing codes of practice for ethical issues arising from genomics

The many ethical issues arising from genomics research need to be debated widely so that individual countries can develop their own frameworks on fundamental principles which have been agreed internationally. It is crucially important that the views of all Member States are represented in these discussions. As has been described, a plethora of national and international bodies have done a great deal of work in supporting the consideration of the ethical implications of these advances, and, for many issues, there is a broad level of agreement about the way forward. For certain key ethical questions, such as the acceptability of research involving human embryonic stem cells, international consensus has yet to be reached and there is still considerable disagreement between different countries and organizations.

As a UN agency committed to promoting human rights and advocacy on behalf of disadvantaged peoples, WHO has an important opportunity to adopt a crucial international leadership role in bioethics, particularly as it relates to the constantly changing issues which will arise as genomics research expands in future years, and the resulting impacts on global health equity. This activity could be focused through the new Ethics in Health initiative, and build on the planning work undertaken by WHO's Ethical, Legal and Social Implications (ELSI) of Genomics Programme over the last two years. Working with other international organizations as appropriate, WHO could use its convening power to facilitate the development of the broad-based codes of practice, and then work actively to promote these principles. Individual Member States can then develop their own ethical frameworks based on these fundamental principles.

Through developing this enhanced role in bioethics and by maintaining close collaborative links with other organizations working in this field, WHO should be in a position to anticipate new ethical issues in this field as they arise and offer well-informed advice and leadership to its Member States. Finally, to ensure a sustainable bioethics programme at WHO, it should receive a core budget and not be left to rely on extra-budgetary funding.

7. Development of regulatory principles and capacities to safeguard against the risks and hazards of genomics research and its applications

Genomics is evolving and opening up a new and completely unexplored technology, which presents a number of potential risks and hazards to public safety and the environment. All Member States must establish regulatory frameworks to monitor and control the commercial and medical application of genomics research in the public interest. Many of the countries in which clinical genetics, recombinant DNA technology and biotechnology are not yet established, or are in the early stages of development, do not have appropriate regulatory structures in place, either at a national level or within individual research institutions. Effective regulatory mechanisms are now well-established in many developed countries and the procedures for setting them up are clearly defined. Member States which are in the process of establishing DNA technologies should consider and build on these principles in establishing their own regulatory mechanisms.

WHO could play an important role in providing advice and assistance to its Member States to enable them to establish simple regulatory systems for the wide variety of technologies that are being developed from genomics based on these recognized principles. WHO could also play a leading role in working with other international organizations and its Member States to harmonize regulatory principles for safeguarding the risks of these new technologies, as they emerge. Where sufficient expertise is not available, WHO could provide technical cooperation to Member States to help to develop local training programmes in this important field. Again, there are major opportunities for fostering local networking and developed-developing country cooperation to further this goal.

10.2.3 An Advocacy Role for WHO

8. Advocating a balance between well-tried research methodology and genomics research

Given the uncertainties regarding current predictions for the health care benefits that may result from this new and rapidly developing field and the time-scales involved, it is crucial that all Member States maintain a balance between genomics and more conventional and well-tried approaches of clinical research, epidemiology and public health. Indeed, as has been stressed throughout this Report, genomics will only fulfil its health care potential if it is integrated alongside these more traditional and well- established fields.

In a global context, there is a danger that genomics research in the more developed countries will become increasingly directed at their own health care problems, particularly as such a high proportion of this work is being driven by commercial interests. There is widespread concern that there is already a rapidly escalating imbalance in these countries between support for genomics research targeted to their particular health priorities, and branches of medical research that are critical for improving health in the developing world, including epidemiology, public health, health demography, and primary care. Increasingly high-technology approaches of the postgenome era are likely to magnify this inequality still further. It is crucial that to redress existing global inequalities in health, developed countries spend more, rather than less on these research fields. Member States must ensure that support for genomics is not having a deleterious effect on funding and recruitment for these more traditional disciplines, which will often have more immediate application to developing countries.

It is vital that WHO advocates the maintenance of a relevant balance in research, development and health care provision between these well-tried research fields and work directed at the medical applications of genomics, both in the context of individual Member States and at a global level.

9.   Ensuring that the medical advances from genomics are accessible to the developing countries

It is likely that many of the health care products and technologies that result from genomics will, at least at first, be very expensive, and as a result might not be accessible to the world's poor. The inevitable consequence would be an increase in health care disparities both within and between countries. As is discussed in detail in Section 7, a key concern that was raised by the vast majority of the individuals and organizations that were consulted in the preparation of this Report is that current practices in the management of intellectual property, particularly the granting of patents on fundamental genomic information, will accentuate these inequalities still further.

The lack of international consensus regarding the status of patents on gene sequences and other genomic elements is a critical problem, and there is a major concern that the granting of such patents will substantially restrict the ability of developing countries to access the fruits of genomics research and apply these to local health care priorities.

Many countries are developing and establishing their own patenting laws, and attempts to develop internationally applicable principles, such as the WTO TRIPS Agreement and the 1998 European Biotechnology Directive, raise many worrying issues, not least the wisdom of applying the patent laws of the developed nations to the developing world. This deeply unsatisfactory situation is compounded by escalating concerns that large transnational corporations are becoming more powerful than many governments and have greater lobbying power. It is clear that if the fruits of genomics are to be developed for medical care, companies will require patent protection for their inventions. However, the current situation has gone too far in terms of promulgating a culture of ownership, and if it is allowed to continue it will inevitably lead to further inequalities in global health care. All Member States should increase efforts to consider the implications of current intellectual property practices on global health issues as a matter of urgency.

Given the critical importance of resolving this issue in the interests of world health, it is crucial that WHO adopts a proactive role as advocate for health equity in international debates on intellectual property issues. In order for it to undertake this role, it will need to form a clear policy position on these issues. This might require the development of a critical mass of internal expertise and might be assisted by the establishment of an expert working group to examine the current situation regarding the patenting of DNA and its products. Such a group could then develop principles upon which patent laws should be reconsidered so that they do not lead to further inequalities in health care. In formulating WHO policy on this issue, it might be appropriate to place this issue on the agenda of the World Health Assembly at a suitable time.

10. Advocating increased investment in genomics research and development directed at the health problems of developing countries

It should be more widely recognized that the health problems of the developing world, including both communicable and non-communicable diseases, are global concerns. Indeed, the increasing trend towards globalization means that diseases which have hitherto been localized to these countries will increasingly impact on developed countries. It is clear that there is a critical need for greater investment at a global level in research and development activities focused at these diseases.

It is crucial that the potential of genomics for the development of new approaches for the control and management of such diseases is realized. Many Member States in the developing world will need to build their own capacity for genomics research and downstream biotechnology research and development to enable them to participate actively and move forward in this field. This process may be facilitated through the types of regional and developed-developing country partnerships described above. However, for other Member States, investment in genomics research might not constitute an immediate priority relative to others for improving their health status at this stage. To ensure the equitable application of genomics research to global health needs, it is clear that there must be enhanced support for research and development programmes targeted to the health problems of the developing world by public, not-for-profit, and private research funders in countries in which genomics technology is well-established.

There is a clear role for WHO in advocating an increase in the availability of resources for genomics research targeted to the health needs of developing countries.

11. Promoting educational and public engagement programmes for the genomics era

Societies need to be better prepared for the medical application of genomics and its consequences. There is a crucial need for all Member States to improve awareness and understanding of genetics in general, and the medical potential of genomics in particular, not just among the general public, but also among government officers, health service administrators, the media and the medical profession itself.

In this new era, educational programmes at all levels will be required to communicate these concepts effectively. It is vital that schoolchildren are introduced to the principles of genetics and ethics, and the inclusion of these subjects in educational curricula and improving the standards of science teaching constitute key priorities. Effective mechanisms are also needed to communicate these ideas to the general public, and the development of a well-informed media will be important in this regard. These approaches should enable policy-makers to engage the public in an informed two-way dialogue to guide the development of ethical and regulatory systems. The development of mechanisms for facilitating public debate will be essential to foster public confidence in these policy frameworks.

To prepare its health sectors for genomics, Member States must ensure that genetics becomes an integral component of medical education, and of continuing training programmes for physicians, nurses and other health workers. Member States should also consider developing educational activities in the technology and ethical implications of genomics for health service administrators and other policy-makers. They should explore regional and other collaborative approaches for the establishment of these programmes, as appropriate.

WHO advocacy will be important in improving knowledge of genetics and genomics at every level — in schools, among the public, in medical education, in health care administration and in government. WHO could provide technical assistance and advice to aid Member States in establishing educational and public engagement programmes.

10.3   CLOSING SUMMARY AND KEY MESSAGES

Although the current applications of genomics for day-to-day clinical practice are very limited, and it is difficult to predict the extent to which they will change medical care or when this will happen, there is no doubt that genetics will assume an increasingly important role in medical research and health care over the next few decades. It is essential that, as this field evolves, the developing countries do not get left behind.

This Report has attempted to give advice on how, without a major increase in expenditure but by improved organization, clinical genetics can be used immediately to introduce the technology of genomics into the developing countries. Following its introduction, this technology may then be adapted to their immediate needs, in the fields of communicable disease and the inherited anaemias, for example. The remainder of the Report suggests how WHO can assist the governments of its Member States in preparing for the clinical, biotechnological, regulatory and ethical requirements of the genomics era while, at the same time, maintaining a balance of research and development between this new field and the well-tried approaches of medical research and practice.

It is suggested that this completely new field of biological science has enormous potential for improving health care, but that there are still many doubts and uncertainties about if and when these advances will materialize. Consequently, a cautious and balanced, double-edged approach to health care planning offers WHO and its Member States the most appropriate way forward for the era of genomics research.

ANNEX A *Glossary of Technical Terms*

Algorithm: In computational terminology, a programme designed to perform a specific calculation or problem-solving function.

Allele: An alternative form of a gene at the same chromosomal locus.

Amino acid: The constituent subunits of proteins. Amino acids polymerize to form linear chains linked by peptide bonds; such chains are termed polypeptides. There are twenty naturally occurring amino acids of which all proteins are made.

Antibody: A protein produced by the immune system in response to an antigen (a molecule that is perceived to be foreign). Antibodies bind specifically to their target antigen to help the immune system destroy the foreign entity.

Autosome: Any chromosome other than a sex chromosome.

Base: *See nucleotide base*

Bacterial artificial chromosome (BAC): DNA vectors into which large DNA fragments can be inserted and cloned in a bacterial host.

Bioinformatics: The discipline encompassing the development and utilization of computational facilities to store, analyse and interpret biological data.

Biotechnology: The industrial application of biological processes, particularly recombinant DNA technology and genetic engineering.

Blastocyst: The mammalian embryo at the stage at which it is implanted into the wall of the uterus.

Carrier: A person who is heterozygous, that is carries one allele, for a recessive disease, and hence does not display the disease phenotype but can pass it on to the next generation.

Cell Cycle: The term given to the series of tightly regulated steps that a cell goes through between its creation and its division to form two daughter cells.

Chromosome: Subcellular structures which convey the genetic material of an organism.

Clone: A line of cells derived from a single cell and therefore carrying identical genetic material.

Cloning vector: A small circle of DNA (plasmid) or modified bacterio-phage (bacterial virus) that can carry a segment of foreign DNA into an appropriate host organism (e.g. a bacterial, yeast or mammalian cell). Used to amplify the amount of foreign DNA or for generating its protein product.

Comparative genomics: The comparison of genome structure and function across different species in order to further understanding of biological mechanisms and evolutionary processes.

Complementary DNA (cDNA): DNA generated from an expressed messenger RNA through a process known as reverse transcription.

Congenital: Any trait, condition or disorder that exists from birth.

Cytoplasm: The internal matrix of a cell. The cytoplasm is the area between the outer periphery of a cell (the cell membrane) and the nucleus (in a eukaryotic cell).

Demographic transition: As used in this Report, the change in a society from extreme poverty to a stronger economy, often associated by a transition in the pattern of diseases from malnutrition and infection to the intractable conditions of middle and old age, cardiovascular disease, diabetes, and cancer, for example.

DNA (deoxyribonucleic acid): The chemical that comprises the genetic material of all cellular organisms.

DNA cloning: Replication of DNA sequences ligated into a suitable vector in an appropriate host organism (see also Cloning vector).

DNA sequencing: Technologies through which the order of base pairs in a DNA molecule can be determined.

Dominant: An allele is described as dominant if it exerts its phenotypic effect when present in the heterozygous state.

Enzyme: An enzyme is a biological catalyst: a protein which controls the rate of a biochemical reaction within a cell.

Eukaryote: An organism whose cells show internal compartmentalization in the form of membrane-bounded organelles (includes animals, plants, fungi and algae).

Exon: The sections of a gene that code for all of its functional product. Eukaryotic genes may contain many exons interspersed with non-coding introns.

Expressed sequence tag (EST): Partial or full complementary DNA sequences which can serve as markers for regions of the genome which encode expressed products.

Founder effect: Changes in allelic frequencies that occur when a small group is separated from a large population and establishes a colony in a new location.

Functional genomics: The development and implementation of technologies to characterize the mechanisms through which genes and their products function and interact with each other and with the environment.

Gene: The fundamental unit of heredity. In molecular terms, a gene comprises a length of DNA that encodes a functional product, which may be a polypeptide (a whole or constituent part of a protein) or a ribonucleic acid.

Genetics: The study of heredity.

Gene expression: The process through which a gene is activated at particular time and place so that its functional product is produced.

Gene therapy: The introduction of genetic material into an individual, or the modification of the individual's genetic material, in order to achieve a therapeutic objective.

Genetic code: The relationship between the order of nucleotide bases in the coding region of a gene and the order of amino acids in the polypeptide product. It is a universal, triplet, non-overlapping code such that each set of three bases (termed a codon) specifies which of the 20 amino acids is present in the polypeptide chain product at a particular position.

Genetic counselling: A process through which patients who are at risk from genetic disease are provided with accurate information about a particular genetic test and the implications of the results in a non-directive manner.

Genetic epidemiology: A field of research in which correlations are sought between phenotypic trends and genetic variation across population groups.

Genetic map: A map showing the positions of genetic markers along the length of a chromosome relative to each other (genetic map) or in absolute distances from each other (physical map).

Genetic susceptibility: Predisposition to a particular disease due to the presence of a specific allele or combination of alleles in an individual's genome.

Genome: The sum total of the genetic material present in a particular organism. This includes both the DNA present in the chromosomes and that in subcellular organelles (e.g. mitochondria or chloroplasts). It also includes the RNA genomes of some viruses.

Genome annotation: The process through which landmarks in a genomic sequence are characterized through computational and other means — for example, genes are identified, predictions made as to the function of their products, their regulatory regions defined and intergenic regions characterized.

Genomics: The study of the genome and its action.

Genotype: The total genetic constitution of an organism.

Germ-line cells: A cell with a haploid chromosome content (also referred to as a gamete); in animals, sperm or egg, in plants, pollen or ovum.

Haemoglobin: The molecule in red blood cells which transports oxygen from the lungs to body tissues.

Haplotype: A series of closely linked loci on a chromosome which tend to be inherited together as a block.

Heterozygote: With respect to a particular gene at a defined chromosomal locus, a heterozygote has a different allelic form of the gene on each of the two homologous chromosomes.

Homozygote: With respect to a particular gene at a defined chromosomal locus, a homozygote has the same allelic form of the gene on each of the two homologous chromosomes.

Hormone: A molecule secreted by a cell or tissue in an organism, which has a functional consequence in other cells located remotely.

Human Genome Project: A programme to determine the sequence of the entire three billion (3×10^9) bases of the human genome.

Intron: A non-coding sequence within eukaryotic genes which separates the exons (coding regions). Introns are spliced out of the messenger RNA molecule created from a gene after transcription, prior to translation (protein synthesis).

Knock-out: A technique used primarily in mouse genetics to inactivate a particular gene in order to define its function.

Library: A collection of genomic or complementary DNA sequences from a particular organism that have been cloned in a vector and grown in an appropriate host organism (e.g. bacteria, yeast).

Linkage: The phenomenon whereby pairs of genes which are located in close proximity on the same chromosome tend to be co-inherited.

Locus: The specific site on a chromosome at which a particular gene or other DNA landmark is located.

Marker: A specific feature at an identified physical location on a chromosome, whose inheritance can be followed. The position of a gene implicated in a particular phenotypic effect can be defined through its linkage to such markers.

Meiosis: A process of two successive cell divisions which results in the production of four daughter cells which each contain half the quantity of chromosomal material present in the parent cell. This form of cell division is used to produce gametes in sexually reproducing organisms.

Mendelian inheritance: The pattern of heritability of a particular phenotypic trait that follows the laws of inheritance developed by Mendel. Monogenic disorders or traits show Mendelian inheritance.

Microarray: A grid of nucleic acid molecules of known composition linked to a solid substrate, which can be probed with total messenger RNA from a cell or tissue to reveal changes in gene expression relative to a control sample. Microarray technology, which is also known as "DNA chip" technology, allows the expression of many thousands of genes to be assessed in a single experiment.

Mitochondria: Cellular organelles present in eukaryotic organisms which enable aerobic respiration, which generates the energy to drive cellular processes. Each mitochondria contains a small amount of DNA encoding a small number of genes (approximately 50).

Mitosis: Standard cell division through which a cell divides to produce two daughter cells with identical chromosomal complement to the parent cell.

Model organism: An experimental organism in which a particular physiological process or disease has similar characteristics to the corresponding process in humans, permitting the investigation of the common underlying mechanisms. Models for human diseases (particularly in mice) have been identified through naturally occurring mutations and can be created using sophisticated transgenics technologies.

Molecular biology: The study of biological processes at the molecular level.

Monogenic disease: A disease whose pathology results from the presence of a particular allele of a gene, either in a heterozygous or homozygous state

Multifactorial (multigenic) disease: A disease whose pathology is dependent on the complex interplay of several genetic and environmental factors.

Mutation: A structural change in a DNA sequence resulting from uncorrected errors during DNA replication.

Nucleotide (nucleotide base): Nucleotides are the subunits from which DNA and RNA molecules are assembled. A nucleotide is a base molecule (i.e. adenine, cytosine, guanine and thymine in the case of DNA), linked to a sugar molecule and phosphate groups.

Oncogene: An acquired mutant form of a gene which acts to transform a normal cell into a cancerous one.

Pharmacogenomics: The identification of the genes which influence individual variation in the efficacy or toxicity of therapeutic agents, and the application of this information in clinical practice.

Phenotype: The observable characteristics of an organism.

Physical map: A map showing the absolute distances between genes (see gene mapping).

Plasmid: Circular extra-chromosomal DNA molecules present in bacteria and yeast. Plasmids replicate autonomously each time a bacterium divides and are transmitted to the daughter cells. DNA segments are commonly cloned using plasmid vectors.

Polymerase chain reaction (PCR): A molecular biology technique developed in the mid-1980s through which specific DNA segments may be amplified selectively.

Polymorphism: The stable existence of two or more variant allelic forms of a gene within a particular population, or among different populations.

Positional cloning: The technique through which candidate genes are located in the genome through their co-inheritance with linked markers. It allows genes to be identified for which there is no information regarding the biochemical action of their functional product.

Post-transcriptional modification: A series of steps through which protein molecules are biochemically modified within a cell following their synthesis by translation of messenger RNA. A protein may undergo a complex series of modifications in different cellular compartments before its final functional form is produced.

Pre-implantation genetic diagnosis: Genetic testing on embryos created by in vitro fertilization, with a view to implanting those which do not contain a particular disease gene.

Prenatal diagnosis: Clinical diagnostic techniques to genetically test a developing fetus.

Prokaryote: An organism or cell lacking a nucleus and other membrane bounded organelles. Bacteria are prokaryotic organisms.

Protein: Proteins are biological effector molecules encoded by an organism's genome. A protein consists of one or more polypeptide chains of amino acid subunits. The functional action of a protein depends on its three dimensional structure, which is determined by its amino acid composition.

Proteomics: The development and application of techniques to investigate the protein products of the genome and how they interact to determine biological functions.

Recessive: An allele is described as recessive if it has no phenotypic effect in the heterozygous state.

Recombinant DNA technology: The term given to some techniques of molecular biology and genetic engineering which were developed in the early 1970s. In particular, the use of restriction enzymes, which cleave DNA at specific sites, allow sections of DNA molecules to be inserted into plasmid or other vectors and cloned in an appropriate host organism (e.g. a bacterial or yeast cell).

Regulatory sequence: A DNA sequence to which specific proteins bind to activate or repress the expression of a gene.

Reproductive cloning: Techniques aimed at the generation of an organism with an identical genome to an existing organism.

Restriction enzymes: A family of enzymes derived from bacteria that cut DNA at specific sequences of bases.

Ribosome: Subcellular structures which form the catalytic site of protein synthesis. Ribosomes comprise protein and RNA complexes at which amino acid chains are constructed as directed by the sequence of messenger RNA molecules.

RNA (ribonucleic acid): A single stranded nucleic acid molecule comprising a linear chain made up from four nucleotide subunits (A, C, G and U). There are three types of RNA: messenger, transfer and ribosomal.

Sex chromosome: The pair of chromosomes that determines the sex of an organism. There are two sex chromosomes, X and Y. In the vast majority of organisms, males possess an X and a Y chromosome and females two X chromosomes.

Shotgun sequencing: A cloning method in which total genomic DNA is randomly sheared and the fragments ligated into a cloning vector. Sometimes referred to as "shotgun" cloning.

Signal transduction: The molecular pathways through which a cell senses changes in its external environment and changes its gene expression patterns in response.

Single nucleotide polymorphism (SNP): A chromosomal locus at which a single base variation exists stably within populations (typically defined as each variant form being present in at least 1-2% of individuals).

Splicing: The process through which introns are removed from a messenger RNA prior to translation and the exons adjoined.

Stem cell: A cell which has the potential to differentiate into a variety of different cell types depending on the environmental stimuli it receives.

Synteny: Syntenic genes are genes which reside on the same chromosome.

Telomere: The natural end of a chromosome.

Therapeutic cloning: The generation and manipulation of stem cells with the objective of deriving cells of a particular organ or tissue to treat a disease.

Transcription: The process through which a gene is expressed to generate a complementary messenger RNA molecule.

Transcriptome: The total messenger RNA expressed in a cell or tissue at a given point in time.

Transgene: A gene from one source that has been incorporated int the genome of another organism.

Transgenic animal/plant: A fertile animal or plant that carries an introduced gene(s) in its germ-line.

Translation: The process through which a polypeptide chain of amino acid molecules is generated as directed by the sequence of a particular messenger RNA sequence.

Transposon: A mobile nucleic acid element.

Tumour suppressor gene: A gene which serves to protect cells from entering a cancerous state. According to Knudson's "two-hit" hypothesis, both alleles of a particular tumour suppressor gene must acquire a mutation before the cell will enter a transformed state.

Vector: See Cloning vector.

Yeast two-hybrid system: A genetic method for analysing the interactions of proteins.

ANNEX B *Consultation Process*

ANNEX B1: *Outline of Consultation Process and Timeline*

1. In January 2001, the Director-General of WHO requested that the Advisory Committee on Health Research (ACHR) prepare a Report to examine the impact of genomics on world health, with a key focus on developing countries. This Report would aim to provide a "roadmap and vision" for the scientific potential of genomics to effect health care improvements in the developing world and survey the key ethical, legal, economic and social issues raised by genomics research and its application in these countries. It was envisaged that the Report would play a key role in identifying strategic priorities for how WHO could work to ensure that the potential of the genomics revolution for improving world health was maximized, while ensuring that these wider implications and risks are addressed.

2. The ACHR promptly convened an expert consultant team to help prepare the Report, comprising Professor Sir David Weatherall (Oxford University, United Kingdom), Professor Dan Brock (Brown University, USA) and Professor Chee Heng-Leng (Universiti Putra Malaysia, Malaysia).

3. In order to ensure that the views of key stakeholder groups were taken into consideration in developing the content of the Report, three international consultative meetings were held in June and July 2001 at which representatives from such groups were invited to present their perspectives and discuss issues of concern:

   ■ The international *Consultation on the ACHR Report on Genomics and Health* was held at WHO Headquarters in Geneva on 27 June 2001, and brought together the global ACHR Committee and regional ACHR chairs with scientists, clinicians, representatives from major public and private funders of genomics research, health policy-makers, representatives from international organizations with programmes in bioethics, and participants from civil-society groups.

- The *Brasilia Regional Consultation on Genomics and Health* was held from 16–17 July 2001. At this meeting, the views of scientists, policy-makers and key individuals concerned with the ethical, legal and social implications of genomics in the PAHO/AMRO region were sought.
- The *Bangkok Multi-Regional Consultation on Genomics and Health* was held from 23–25 July 2001. This meeting brought together participants from four WHO regions (SEARO, WPRO, AFRO and EMRO), including: scientists, clinicians, ethicists, representatives of key non-governmental organizations and government policy-makers. There was further participation from two countries in the EURO region.

4. Based on the evidence presented by participants at these three consultations and the key consensus points that emerged from the discussions that took place, the consultant team prepared a preliminary draft of the Report between August and September, 2001. Concurrently, a series of interviews were conducted with key staff members at WHO Headquarters, in order to collate their expert perspectives for consideration in the development of the Report.

5. In early October 2001, the draft Report was circulated to the members of the global ACHR, each cluster within WHO Headquarters, and the Directors of each of the six WHO Regional Offices, for comments and feedback.

6. All inputs and feedback were collated for discussion at a special meeting of the global ACHR on 1–2 November 2001, at which the content and recommendations of the Report were finalized. The consultant team and RPC Secretariat then revised the content of the Report to encompass the points agreed at this meeting. The final draft version was then circulated to the 11 members of the global ACHR in December 2001 for final approval.

ANNEX B2: *Consultations*

B2.1   *Consultation on the ACHR Report on Genomics and Health*
        (WHO Headquarters, Geneva 27 June 2001)
Agenda
Date: Wednesday, 27 June, 2001
Venue: Salle B, WHO Headquarters, Geneva, Switzerland
Chair: Mahmoud Fathalla, Chair of the ACHR.
Moderator: Sir David Weatherall.
Rapporteur: David Carr
Opening by David Nabarro, EXD/DGO
Welcoming remarks by Christopher Murray, EXD/EIP
Welcoming remarks by Derek Yach, EXD/NMH
Welcoming remarks by Mahmoud Fathalla, Chair, ACHR,
Presentations: Applications of genomics in developing countries
    Steve Hoffman (Celera Genomics)
    Michael Morgan (Wellcome Trust Genome Centre)
    Christine Debouck (GlaxoSmithKline)
Presentations: Ethical, legal, social aspects of genomics
    Peteris Zilgalvis (Council of Europe)
    Alex Capron (National Bioethics Advisory Commission)
    Abdallah Daar (University of Toronto)
    Peter Whittaker (European Group on Ethics in Science
    and New Technologies)
Presentations: Community, civil society & gender perspectives
    Sigurdur Gudmundsson (Surgeon General, Iceland)
    Gilles de Wildt (People's Health Assembly)
    Chee-Koon Chan (Citizen's Health Initiative)
    Bernadette Modell (London Medical School)
Round Table discussion (Moderator — Sir David Weatherall)
Concluding Remarks — Sir John Sulston
Closing remarks by Chair — Mahmoud Fathalla

List Of Participants
ACHR Members
Mahmoud Fathalla (Chairman)
    Faculty of Medicine
    Assiut University Hospital, Egypt

Zulfiqar A. Bhutta
    Department of Paediatrics & Child Health
    The Aga Khan University, Pakistan
Barry Bloom
    Harvard School of Public Health, USA
Marian Jacobs*
    Child Health Unit
    Rondebosch, South Africa
Gerald Keusch
    Fogarty International Center
    National Institutes of Health, USA
Maxime Schwartz
    Institut Pasteur, France
Gita Sen*
    Indian Institute of Management
    Bangalore, India
Fumimaro Takaku
    Jichi Medical School, Japan
Cesar G. Victora
    Curso de Pos-Graduaçao em Epidemiologia
    Universidade Federal de Pelotas, Brazil
Lars Walloe
    Department of Physiology
    University of Oslo, Norway
Judith Whitworth
    John Curtin School of Medical Research, Australia
*unable to attend

Regional ACHR Chairs
Petros Beyene
    AACHRD (AFRO), Ethiopia
Jorge E. Allende
    Instituto de Ciencias Biomedicas
    Universidade de Chile, Chile
Nirmal K. Ganguly
    Indian Council of Medical Research, India

Temporary Advisers

Dan Brock
  Center for Biomedical Ethics
  Brown University, USA
Alexander Capron
  Pacific Center for Health Policy and Ethics. University of Southern
  California, USA
David Carr
  Policy Unit
  The Wellcome Trust, UK
Chan Chee Khoon
  School of Social Sciences
  Universiti Sains Malaysia, Malaysia
Chee Heng Leng
  Faculty of Medicine & Health Sciences
  Universiti Putra Malaysia, Malaysia
Abdallah S.Daar
  University of Toronto Joint Centre for Bioethics,, Canada
Christine Debouck
  Worldwide Genomics
  GlaxoSmithKline, USA
Gilles de Wildt
  The People's Health Assembly, UK
Richard Feachem
  Institute for Global Health, USA
G. Feger
  Department of Genomics,
  Institut Serono, Switzerland
Sigurdur Gudmundsson,
  Surgeon General of Iceland,
  Rekjavik, Iceland
John B. Hannum
  Dept of Government Affairs and Public Policy
  GlaxoSmithKline, UK
Stephen Hoffman
  Celera Genomics, USA
Delon Human
  The World Medical Association, France

Klaus Lindpaintner
  Roche Genetics
  F. Hoffman-La-Roche, Switzerland
Alex Mauron
  Unité de recherche et d'enseignement en bioéthique,
  Centre Medical Universitaire, Switzerland
Bernadette Modell
  Royal Free & University College
  London Medical School, UK
Michael Morgan
  The Wellcome Trust, UK
Sir John Sulston
  The Sanger Centre
  Wellcome Trust Genome Campus, UK
Sir David J. Weatherall
  Weatherall Institute of Molecular Medicine
  John Radcliffe Hospital
  Oxford University, UK
Peter Whittaker
  Member of the European Group for Ethics in Science and the New
  Technologies
  National University of Ireland, Ireland
Sebastian Wanless
  Bioethics Committee
  Bristol-Myers Squibb Pharmaceutical Research Institute,
  Princeton, USA
Peteris Zilgalvis,
  Bioethics Division I — Legal Affairs
  Council of Europe
  Strasbourg, France

Observers
Tore Godal
  Global Alliance for Vaccines and Immunisation
  UNICEF, Switzerland
Orio Ikebe
  Department of Philosophy, Human Sciences, Ethics of Science &
  Technology
  UNESCO, France

Roger Kampf
    European Commission
    Permanent Delegation to the International Organizations in
    Geneva, Switzerland
Miguel Gonzalez-Block
    Alliance for Health Policy and Systems Research
    WHO, Switzerland
Sev Fluss
    The Council for International Organizations of Medical Sciences,
    Switzerland
Louis Currat
    Global Forum for Health Research, Switzerland
Andres de Francisco
    Global Forum for Health Research, Switzerland

WHO Staff
Regional Offices
David Okello (WHO Regional Office for Africa)
Alberto Pellegrini (WHO Regional Office for the Ameicas)
Javid Hashmi (representing WHO Regional Office for the
    Eastern Mediterranean)
Yves Charpak (WHO Regional Office for Europe)
Adik Wibowo (WHO Regional Office for South-East Asia)
Chen Ken (WHO Regional Office for the Western Pacific)

WHO Headquarters
Ala Alwan (Management of Noncommunicable Diseases)
Victor Boulyjenkov (Management of Noncommunicable Diseases)
Graeme A.Clugston (Nutrition for Health & Development)
Christine Encrenaz (Essential Drugs & Medicines Policy)
Olivier Fontaine (Child & Adolescent Health)
Elwyn Griffiths (Vaccines & Biologicals)
Richard Helmer (Protection of the Human Environment)
David Heymann (Communicable Diseases)
Ayoade Oduola (Special Programme for Research & Training in Tropical
    Diseases)
Carlos Morel (Special Programme for Research & Training in Tropical
    Diseases)
Christopher Murray (Evidence & Information for Policy)

David Nabarro (Director General's Office)
Lembit Rago (Essential Drugs & Medicines Policy)
Jorgen Schlundt (Protection of the Human Environment)
Johannes Sommerfeld (Special Programme for Research & Training in Tropical Diseases)
Sergio Spinaci (Evidence & Information for Policy)
Kathleen Strong (Management of Noncommunicable Diseases)
Hans Troedsson (Child & Adolescent Health)
Paul van Look (Reproductive Health & Research)
Daniel Wikler (Evidence for Health Policy)
Derek Yach (Noncommunicable Diseases & Mental Health)

RPC (Research Policy & Cooperation) SECRETARIAT
Nicole Biros
Danièle Doebeli
Elsa Fre Kidane
Takeo Imai
Marissa Khomin
Tikki Pang
Patricia Picard
Abha Saxena
Sacha Sidjanski

B2.2   *Brasilia Regional Consultation on Genomics and World Health (Brasilia, 16–17 July 2001)*
List of Participants
Alexandre Mauron
    Unit de researche et d'enseignment en bioethique
    Centre Medical Universitaire, Switzerland
Ana Alice Da Costa E Silva
    A&C Eventos, Promocoes e Consultoria, Brazil
Beatriz H. Tess
    Department of Science and Technology
    Ministry of Health, Brazil
César Jacoby
    Department of Science and Technology
    Ministry of Health, Brazil

Corina Bontempo Duca De Freitas
  Comissao Nacional de Etica em Pesquisa
  Ministry of Health, Brazil
Euzenir Nunes Sarno
  Pesquisa e Desenvolvimento Technologico
  Fundacao Oswaldo Cruz, Brazil
Fernando Lolas
  Programa Regional de Bioetica
  OPS/OMS, Chile
Gerald T. Keusch
  Fogarty International Center
  National Institutes of Health, USA
Imogen Evans
  Medical Research Council, UK
Jacobo Finkelman
  Representate da OPAS/OMS no Brazil, Brazil
José Escamilla
  OPAS/OMS, Brazil
José Maria Cantu
  University of Guadalajara, Mexico
Leocir Pessini
  Universidade Sao Camilo, Brazil
Lorenzo Agar Corbinos
  Universidad de Chile
  Programa Regional de Bioetica, Chile
Lucia Aleixo
  Departmentio de Cienca e Tecnologia em Saude
  Ministry of Health, Brazil
Volnei Garrafa
  Bioetica da Universidade de Brasilia, Brazil
Victor B. Penchaszadeh
  WHO Collaborating Center for Community Genetics and Education
  Beth Israel Medical Center, Albert Einstein College of Medicine, USA
Zuleica Portela Albuquerque
  Consultora em Nutricao e Coordenacao De Investigacoes e Availicao
  de Tecnologias
  OPAS/OMS, Brazil

B2.3   *The Bangkok Multiregional Consultation on Genomics and World Health (23–25 July 2001)*

Agenda

Monday, 23 July 2001

Welcome Address
        Prawase Wasi (National Health Foundation)
Brief Presentation on the Objectives of the Meeting
        Tikki Pang (WHO, Geneva)
Plenary Session I: An Overview of Genomics and Health: Implications for Developing Countries
        Sir David Weatherall
Plenary Session II: ELSI Implications from the Perspective of Developing Countries
        Chee Heng-Leng
General Discussion: Regional Perspective on Genomics and Health: WHO Regional Office for the Eastern Mediterranean
        Abdallah Daar
Regional Perspective on Genomics and Health: WHO Regional Office for Western Pacific
        Huan-Ming Yang
Discussion
Regional Perspective on Genomics and Health: WHO Regional Office for Africa
        Patrice Matchaba
Genomics and Health: An NGO Perspective
        Seri Psongphit
General Discussion

Tuesday, 24 July 2001

Summary of First Day Meeting
        David Carr
Regional Perspective on Genomics and Health: WHO Regional Office for South East Asia
        Prawase Wasi
Discussion
Developing a Strategic Plan for WHO in the Ethical, Legal and Social Implications of Genomics
        Kathleen Strong
Non-Human Genome Sequences (Pathogens and Vectors)
        John Mattick

Human Genomics and Health Policy
> Mae Wan Ho
Discussion
Group Discussion I — Developing Countries and Genomics Research
> (Introduction by Sangkot Marzuki)
Presentation of Group Work
Group Discussion II — Research Partnerships and Issues Related to
Intellectual Property in Genomics Research (Introduction by Prasit
Palittapongarnpim)
Presentation of Group Work

Wednesday, 25 July 2001
Summary of Second Day Meeting
> David Carr
Group Discussion III — Genetic Testing and Social and Ethical
Implications (Introduction by Chan Chee Khoon)
Presentation of Group Work
Group Discussion IV — Reproductive Health Policy and Advances in
Genomics
Presentation of Group Work
Wrapping Up
> Sir David Weatherall, Tikki Pang and Somsak Chunharas

List of Participants
Sakarindr Bhumiratana
> National Science and Technology Development Agency, Thailand
Vichai Boonsaeng
> Mahidol University, Thailand
David Carr
> The Wellcome Trust, UK
Chan Chee Khoon
> Epidemiology and Health Policy,
> Development Studies Programme,
> Universiti Sains Malaysia, Malaysia
Chee Heng-Leng
> Department of Community Health,
> Faculty of Medicine and Health Sciences,
> Universiti Putra Malaysia, Malaysia

Numkang Chaiput
  National Center For Genetic Engineering and Biotechnology,
  Thailand
Komatra Chuengsathiensab
  Health Policy and Planning Bureau
  Ministry of Public Health, Thailand
Somsak Chunharas
  National Health Foundation, Thailand
Suttikan Chunsuttiwat
  National Health Foundation, Thailand
Jo Cooper
  Centre for Health Law, Ethics and Policy
  University of Newcastle, Australia
Abdallah Daar
  University of Toronto Joint Centre for Bioethics, Canada
K.C.S. Dalpatadu
  Ministry of Health and Indigenous Medicine, Sri Lanka
Nares Damrongchai
  National Center for Genetic Engineering and Biotechnology, Thailand
Kairat Davletov,
  Division of Medico-Social and Preventive Programmes
  National Centre for Health Lifestyle, Kazakhstan
Jade Donavanik
  National Science and Technology Development Agency, Thailand
Du Zhizheng
  International Research Centre for Humanistic and Social Medicine
  Dalian Medical University, People's Republic of China
Suthat Fucharoen
  Thalassemia Research Center
  Mahidol University, Thailand
Norio Fujiki,
  Emeritus Professor, Fukui Medical School, Japan
Mohamed H.A. Hassan
  Third World Academy of Sciences, Italy
Mae-Wan Ho
  Institute of Science in Society, UK
U Htay-Aung
  Department of Medical Research (Upper Myanmar), Myanmar

Amar Jesani,
    Centre for Equity into Health Allied Themes, India
Rossukhon Kangvallert
    Bureau of Health Policy and Planning
    Ministry of Public Health, Thailand
Kiniviliame Keteca
    Fiji Law Reform Commission, Fiji
Azad Khan
    Diabetic Association of Bangladesh, Bangladesh
Vaidutis Kucinskas,
    Human Genetics Centre
    Santriskiu Clinics of Vilnius University Hospital, Lithuania
Liliana Kurniawan,
    Research and Development Centre
    Ministry of Health and Social Welfare, Indonesia
Jerzy Leowski
    WHO Regional Office for South East Asia, India
Lim Li Lin
    Third World Network, Malaysia
A.Λ. Loedin
    Indonesian Academy of Sciences
    Commission for Medical Sciences, Indonesia
Lye Munn Sann
    Medical Research Institute, Ministry of Health, Malaysia
Preeda Malasit
    Mahidol University, Thailand
Patrice Matchaba
    Novartis, South Africa
John Mattick
    The Institute for Molecular Bioscience
    University of Queensland, Australia
Phelix Majiwa
    International Livestock Research Institute (ILRI), Nairobi, Kenya
Sangkot Marzuki
    Eijkman Institute for Molecular Biology, Indinesia
Na Doe Sun
    Department of Biochemistry
    University of Ulsan College of Medicine, South Korea

Sumalee Nimmannit
Faculty of Medicine, Siriraj Hospital,
Mahidol University, Thailand
Chantana Padungtod
Ministry of Public Health, Thailand
Prasit Palittapongarnpim
National Centre for Genetic Engineering and Biotechnology, Thailand
Tikki Pang
WHO Headquarters, Switzerland
Vichan Panich
Thailand Research Fund, Thailand
Maude Phipps
Department of Allied Health Sciences
University of Malaya, Malaysia
Seri Phongphit
The Village Foundation, Thailand
Samlee Pliangbangchang
College of Public Health
Chulalongkorn University, Thailand
Pakdee Potthisiri
Ministry of Public Health, Thailand
Asri Rasad
Yarsi University, Jakarta, Indonesia
Narumol Sawanpanyalert
Ministry of Public Health, Thailand
Kathleen Strong
WHO Headquarters, Switzerland
Chitr Sitti-Amorn
College of Public Health,
Chulalongkorn University, Thailand
Lalji Singh
Centre for Cell and Molecular Biology (CCMB)
Hyderabad, India
Teparkum Sirisak
National Centre for Genetic Engineering and Biotechnology, Thailand
Soe Thien
Department of Medical Research, Myanmar
Herawati Sudoyo
Eijkman Institute for Molecular Biology, Indonesia

Sri Astuti Suparmanto,
  NIHRD Ministry of Health, Indonesia
U Than Sein
  WHO South East Asia Regional Office, India
Thanapaisal Thippayawan
  National Centre For Genetic Engineering and Biotechnology,
  Thailand
U Tun Pe
  Department of Medical Research (Lower Mayanmar), Myanmar
Tan Tun Sein
  Department of Medical Research, Myanmar
I. C. Verma
  Dept of Genetic Medicine
  Sir Ganga Ram Hospital, India
Satupaitea Viali
  Tupea Tomasese Meaole Hospital, Samoa
Pramuan Virutamasen
  Chulalongkorn University, Thailand
Tissa Vitarana
  Advisor, Ministry of Science & Technology, Sri Lanka
Wanchai Wanachiwanawin
  Faculty of Medicine, Siriraj Hospital
  Mahidol University, Thailand
Prawase Wasi
  Mahidol University, Thailand
Sir David Weatherall
  Weatherall Institute of Molecular Medicine
  Oxford University, UK
Prapon Wilairat
  Faculty of Science
  Mahidol University, Thailand
Sidong Xiong
  The Center for Gene Immunisation and Vaccines, People's Republic
  of China
Huanming Yang
  Human Geneome Center, People's Republic of China
C.A.K Yesudian
  Tata Institute of Social Sciences, India

Yongyuth Yuthavong
    Thailand Institute of Science and Technology
    National Science and Technology Development Agency, Thailand
Zainul F. Zainuddin
    School of Health Sciences
    Universiti Sains Malaysia, Malaysia

ANNEX B3: *List of Contributing WHO Staff*

WHO Headquarters
Ala Alwan (Management of Noncommunicable Diseases)
Anarfi Asamoa-Baah (External Relations & Governing Bodies)
Robert Beaglehole (Health & Development)
Ruth Bonita (Noncommunicable Diseases Surveillance)
Victor Boulyjenkov (Management of Noncommunicable Diseases)
Catherine D'Arcangues (Reproductive Health & Research)
Boris Dobrokhotov (Special Programme for Research & Training in
    Tropical Diseases)
Christopher Dye (Stop TB Programme)
Christine Encrenaz (Essential Drugs & Medicines Policy)
Jose Esparza (UNAIDS/WHO HIV Vaccine Inititive)
David Griffin (Reproductive Health & Research)
David Heymann (Communicable Diseases)
Ann Kern (Sustainable Development & Healthy Environments)
Janis Lazdins-Helds (Special Programme for Research & Training in
    Tropical Diseases)
Shanthi Mendis (Management of Noncommunicable Diseases)
Maristela Monteiro (Mental Health & Substance Dependence)
Carlos Morel (Special Programme for Research & Training in Tropical
    Diseases)
Christopher Murray (Evidence & Information for Policy)
David Nabarro (Director General's Office)
Ayoade Oduola (Special Programme for Research & Training in Tropical
    Diseases)
Lembit Rägo (Essential Drugs & Medicines Policy)
Eva Sandborg (Management of Noncommunicable Diseases)
Shekhar Saxena (Mental Health & Substance Dependence)
Jorgen Schlundt (Protection of the Human Environment)
Maria Sepulveda Bermedo (Management of Noncommunicable Diseases)

Sergio Spinaci (Evidence & Information for Policy)
Johannes Sommerfeld (Special Programme for Research & Training in
   Tropical Diseases)
Kathleen Strong (Management of Noncommunicable Diseases)
Yasuhiro Suzuki (Health Technology & Pharmaceuticals)
Hans Troedsson (Child & Adolescent Health)
Yeya Toure (Special Programme for Research & Training in Tropical
   Diseases)
Paul van Look (Reproductive Health & Research)
Effy Vayena (Reproductive Health & Research)
Daniel Wikler (Evidence for Health Policy)
Derek Yach (Noncommunicable Diseases & Mental Health)

Council for International Organizations of Medical Science (CIOMS)
Sev Fluss
James Gallagher
Juhana Idänpään-Heikkilä

Annex B4: *List of Relevant Background WHO Work on Genetics,
   Genomics and Biotechnology*
*Proposed International Guidelines on Ethical Issues in Medical Genetics and Genetic
   Services* Geneva, World Health Organization 1998. (document
   WHO/HGN/GL/ETH/98.1)
   (Website http://whqlibdoc.who.int/hq/1998/WHO_HGN_GL_ETH_98.1.pdf)
*Statement of the WHO Expert Advisory Group on Ethical Issues in Medical
   Genetic.* WHO Expert Advisory Group on Ethical Issues in Medical Genetics.
   Geneva, World Health Organization
   (document WHO/HGN/ETH/98.2)
Medical Genetic Services in Latin America. Report of a WHO Collaborating Centre
   for Community Genetics and Education. Geneva, World Health Organization
   1998
   (document WHO/HGN/CONS/MGS/98.4)
   (Website http://whqlibdoc.who.int/hq/1998/WHO_HGN_CONS_MGS_98.4.pdf)
*Health Promotion in the Post Genomics Era — Preparing to receive and make good
   use of new genetic knowledge.* Report of a Temporary Advisor. Geneva, World
   Health Organization 1998
   (document WHO/HGN/CONS/98.8)

Services for the Prevention and Management of Genetic Disorders and Birth Defects in Developing Countries. Report of a joint WHO/WAOPBD meeting, The Hague, 5–7 January 1999. Geneva, World Health Organization 1999 (document WHO/HGN/GL/WAOPBD/99.1) (Website http://www.who.int/ncd/hgn/reppub_malta.htm)

Seminar on Biotechnology and Its Impact on Human Health. Frontiers in Research Program/RPC/99. Geneva, World Health Organization 1999.

Ethical Issues in Genetics, Cloning and Biotechnology: possible future directions for WHO. Report of an informal consultation. Geneva, World Health Organization 1999. (document WHO/EIP/GPE/00.1)

Daar AS, Mattei JF (1999): Medical Genetics and Biotechnology: Implications for Public Health. Annex 1 in *Ethical Issues in Genetics, Cloning and Biotechnology: possible future directions for WHO.* Report of an informal consultation. Geneva, World Health Organization 1999. (document WHO/EIP/GPE/00.1)

Primary Health Care Approaches for Prevention and Control of Congenital and Genetic Disorders. Report of a WHO meeting Cairo, Egypt, 6–8 December 1999. Geneva, World Health Organization 2000. (document WHO/HGN/WG/00.1) (Website http://www.who.int/ncd/hgn/hcprevention.htm)

Statement of the WHO Expert Consultation on New Developments in Human Genetics. Geneva, World Health Organization 2000. (document WHO/HGN/WG/00.3) (Website http://www.who.int/ncd/hgn/Statement.pdf)

Operational Guidelines for Ethical Committees that Review Biomedical Research. Geneva, World Health Organization 2000. (document TDR/PRD/ETHICS/2000.1)

Work Plan for the ethical, legal and social implications of genetics — a draft for discussion Management of Non-communicable Diseases cluster. Geneva, World Health Organization 2001.

The WHO European Region and the Human Genome — A position paper. Copenhagen, WHO EURO, 2001

Cloning in Human Health — Report by the Director General. Fifty-third World Health Assembly, Geneva, World Health Organization 2000. (document A53/15). (Website http://www.who.int/gb/EB_WHA/PDF/WHA53/ea15.pdf)

Regional Perspectives in Human Genetics, Genomes and Health. New Delhi, WHO SEARO 2001.

Annex B5: *Profiles of Report writers*

Sir David Weatherall is Emeritus Regius Professor of Medicine, and
Honorary Director, Weatherall Institute of Molecular Medicine,
University of Oxford, United Kingdom. He was previously Nuffield
Professor of Clinical Medicine, University of Oxford (1974–1992)
and Professor of Haematology, University of Liverpool (1971–74).
Professor Weatherall's major research contributions, resulting in over
700 publications, have been in the elucidation of the clinical, biochemical and molecular heterogeneity of the thalassaemias and in the
application of this information to the development of programmes for
the prevention of these diseases in different populations throughout
the world. His book, *The New Genetics and Clinical Practice*, is a
widely used textbook in many molecular biology courses. He holds
numerous honours including Knight Bachelor (1987), Commandeur
de l'Ordre de la Couronne (1994), Fellow of the Royal Society
(1977), Foreign Associate, National Academy of Sciences USA (1990)
and numerous honorary degrees and fellowships from universities in
the United Kingdom and elsewhere in the world. In January 2002,
Professor Weatherall was awarded the prestigious Prince Mahidol
Award from the Government of Thailand in recognition of his work
in the field of thalassaemia.

Dan Brock is Charles C.Tillinghast, Jr. University Professor, Professor of
Philosophy and Biomedical Ethics, and Director of the Center for
Biomedical Ethics at Brown University where he has a joint appoint-
ment in the Philosophy Department (of which he was Chair in
1980–86) and in the Medical School. He received his B.A. in economics from Cornell University and his Ph.D. in philosophy from
Columbia University. He served as Staff Philosopher on the
President's Commission for the Study of Ethical Problems in Medicine
in 1981–82. In 1993 he was a member of the Ethics Working Group
of the Clinton Task Force on National Health Reform. He has been a
consultant in biomedical ethics and health policy to numerous national and international bodies, including the Office of Technology
Assessment of the U.S. Congress, the Institute of Medicine, the
National Bioethics Advisory Commission, and the World Health
Organization. He is currently Visiting Senior Scholar in the
Department of Clinical Bioethics at the National Institutes of Health
(2001 2002). He was President of the American Association of

Bioethics in 1995–96, and was a founding Board Member of the American Society for Bioethics and Humanities. He is the author of over 130 published papers in bioethics health policy, and moral and political philosophy, which have appeared in books and leading scholarly journals. Professor Brock is the author of *Deciding For Others: The Ethics of Surrogate Decision Making*, 1989, (with A. Buchanan), *Life and Death: Philosophical Essays in Biomedical Ethics*,1993, and *From Chance to Choice: Genetics and Justice* (with A. Buchanan, N. Daniels and D. Wikler) 2000, all published by Cambridge University Press.

Heng-Leng Chee is an associate professor at the Community Health Department of the Faculty of Medicine and Health Sciences at the Universiti Putra Malaysia. Her research interests are primarily in the field of health care policy and women's health, and she has published on subjects relating to the health care system in Malaysia, community health and nutrition, and women's health and reproductive rights. In 1984, she co-edited a volume entitled *Designer Genes: IQ, Ideology, and Biology*. She has presented papers on various other aspects of bioethics. In 1993–1996, she was a member of the International Bioethics Committee of the United Nations Educational, Scientific and Cultural Organization (UNESCO), in conjunction with which she organized a consultation in Malaysia for contributing comments to the initial process of drafting the international instrument on the protection of the human genome, and also served on the subcommittee for population genetics research. Dr. Chee Heng Leng is actively involved in non-profit organizations, being a founder member of the Women's Development Collective, the All Women's Action Society, as well as the Citizens' Health Initiative, a group that carries out public education and advocacy for a universally accessible health care system that is publicly financed, owned and operated.

ANNEX C *References and Further Reading*

SECTION 2

References

Baker D, Sali A (2001). Protein structure prediction and structural genomics. *Science*, 294:93–96.

Brenner SE (2001). A tour of structural genomics. *Nature Reviews Genetics*, 2:801–809.

Enserink M (2001). Two new steps towards a "better mosquito" *Science*, 293:2370–2371.

Fraser CM, Eisen JA, Salzberg SL (2000). Microbial genome sequencing. *Nature*, 406:799–803.

Hasty J, McMillen D, Isaacs F, Collins JJ (2001). Computational studies of gene regulatory networks: *in numero* molecular biology. *Nature Reviews Genetics*, 2:268–279.

Hoffman SL, Subramanian GM, Collins FH, Venter JC (2002). Plasmodium, human and Anopheles genomics and malaria. *Nature* 415:702–709.

Justice MJ (2000). Capitalizing on large-scale mouse mutagenesis screens. *Nature Reviews Genetics*, 1: 109–115.

Lander ES, Linton LM, Birren B, Nusbaum C, Zody MC, Baldwin J, et al. (2001). Initial sequencing and analysis of the human genome. *Nature*, 409:860–921.

Lockhart DJ, Winzler EA (2000). Genomics, gene expression and DNA arrays. *Nature*, 405:827–836.

Nadeau JH (2001). Modifier genes in mice and humans. *Nature Reviews Genetics*, 2:165–174.

Sachidanandam R, Weissman D, Schmidt SC, Kakol JM, Stein LD, Marth G, et al. (2001). A map of human genome sequence variation containing 1.42 million single nucleotide polymorphisms. *Nature*, 409:928–933.

Singer PA, Daar AS (2001). Harnessing genomics and biotechnology to improve global health equity. *Science*, 294:87–89.

Stein L (2001). Genome annotation: from sequence to biology. *Nature Reviews Genetics*, 2:493–503.

Venter JC, Adams MD, Myers EW, Li PW, Mural RJ, Sutton GG, et al. (2001). The sequence of the human genome. *Science*, 291:1304–1349.

Further Reading

Alberts B, Bray D, Lewis J, Raff M, Watson JD, Roberts K (1994). *The molecular biology of the cell (3rd edition)*. New York and London, Garland Publishing.

Burley SK, Almo SC, Bonanno JB, Capel M, Chance MR, Gaasterland T, et al. (1999). Structural genomics: beyond the human genome project. *Nature Genetics*, 23:151–157.

Claverie JM (1999). Computational methods for the identification of differential and coordinated gene expression. *Human Molecular Genetics*, 8:1821–1832.

Creighton TE (1997). Proteins. In: Dulbecco R (ed) *Encylopedia of Human Biology*. New York, Academic Press, 189–203.

Fields S (2001). Proteomics in Genomeland. *Science*, 291:1221–1224.

Jacob HJ, Kwitek AE (2002) Rat genetics: attaching physiology and pharmacology to the genome. Nature Review Genetics, 3:33–42

Lewin B (1997). *Genes VII*. Oxford, Oxford University Press.

Weatherall DJ (1991). *The New Genetics and Clinical Practice*, 3rd ed. Oxford, Oxford University Press.

SECTION 3

References

Baier LJ, Permana PA, Yang X, Pratley RE, Hanson RL, Shen GQ, et al. (2000). A calpain-10 gene polymorphism is associated with reduced muscle mRNA levels and insulin resistance. *The Journal of Clinical Investigation*, 106:R69–R73.

Barker DJP(ed) (2001). *Fetal origins of cardiovascular and lung disease*. New York, Macel Dekker Inc.

Bojang KA, Milligan PJ, Pinder M, Vigneron L, Alloueche A, Kester KE, et al. (2001). Efficacy of RTS,S/ASO2 malaria vaccine against *Plasmodium falciparum* infection in semi-immune adult men in The Gambia: a randomised trial. *Lancet*, 358:1927–1933.

Druker BJ, Lydon NB (2000). Lessons learned from the development of ab1 tyrosine kinase inhibitor for chronic myelogenous leukaemia. *The Journal of Clinical Investigation*, 105:3–7.

Enserink M (2001). Two new steps towards a "better mosquito." *Science*, 293:2370–2371.

Evans WE, Relling MV (1999). Translating functional genomics into rational therapeutics. *Science*, 286:487–491.

Ferber D (2001). Safer and virus-free? *Science*, 294:1638–1642.

Horikawa Y, Oda N, Cox NJ, Li X, Orho-Melander M, Hara M, et al. (2000). Genetic variation in the gene encoding calpain-10 is associated with type 2 diabetes mellitus. *Nature Genetics*, 26:163–175.

Hugot JP, Chamaillard M, Zouali H, Lesage S, Cezard JP, Belaiche J, et al. (2001). Association of NOD2 leucine-rich repeat variants with susceptibility to Crohn's disease. *Nature*, 411:599–603.

Kaji EH, Leiden JM (2001). Gene and stem cell therapies. *Journal of the American Medical Association*, 285:545–550.

Kwok PY (2001).Genetic association by whole-genome analysis. *Science*, 294:1669–1670.

Lesage S, Zouali H, Colombel JF, Belaiche J, Cézard JP, Tysk C, et al. (2000). Genetic analyses of chromosome 12 loci in Crohn's disease. *Gut*, 47:787–791.

Letvin NL, Bloom BR, Hoffman SL (2001). Prospects for vaccines to protect against AIDS, tuberculosis and malaria. *Journal of the American Medical Association*, 285:606–611.

Livingston DM, Shivdasani R (2001). Towards mechanism-based cancer care. *Journal of the American Medical Association*, 285:588–593.

Novartis Foundation Symposium 235 (2001). *Ageing vulnerability: causes and interventions*. New York, John Wiley & Sons.

Orme IM, McMurray DN, Belisle JT (2001). Tuberculosis vaccine development: recent progress. *Trends in Microbiology*, 9:115–118.

Peltonen L, McKusick VA (2001). Dissecting human disease in the postgenomic era. *Science*, 291:1224–1229

Roses AD (2000). Pharmacogenetics and the practice of medicine. *Nature*, 405:857–865.

Schindler T, Bornmann W, Pellicena P, Miller WT, Clarkson B, Kuriyan J (2000). Structural mechanism for STI-571 inhibition of abelson tyrosine kinase. *Science* 289:1938–1942.

Scriver CR (1995). Review of: assessing genetic risks: implications for health and social policy. *American Journal of Human Genetics*, 56:814–816.

Somia N, Verma IM (2000). Gene therapy: trials and tribulations. *Nature Reviews Genetics* 1:91–99.

WHO (2000). *Statement of the WHO Expert Consultation on New Developments in Human Genetics*. Geneva, World Health Organization, 2000. (document WHO/HGN/WG/00.3)

(Accessed at http://www.who.int/ncd/hgn/Statement.pdf Jan 16, 2002)

Weatherall DJ, Clegg JB(eds) (2001). *The thalassemia syndromes*,4th ed. Oxford, Blackwell Science Publishing Co.

Weatherall DJ (2001). Phenotype genotype relations in monogenic disease: lessons from the thalassaemics. *Nature Reviews, Genetics*, 2:245–255.

Wilson JF, Weale ME, Smith AC, Gratrix F, Fletcher B, Thomas MG, et al. (2001). Population genetic structure of variable drug response. *Nature Genetics*, 29:265–269.

Ye X, Al-Babili S, Kloti A, Zhang J, Lucca P, Beyer P, et al. (2000). Engineering the provitamin A (β-carotene) biosynthetic pathway into (carotenoid-free) rice endosperm. *Science*, 287:303–305.

Further Reading

Ashton PD, Curwen RS, Wilson RA (2001). Linking proteome and genome: how to identify parasite proteins. *Trends in Parasitology* 17(4):198–202.

Bloom BR (2000). On the particularity of pathogens. *Nature*, 406:760–761.

Brack C, Lithgow G, Osiewacz H, Toussaint O (2000). EMBO workshop report: molecular and cellular gerontology. *EMBO Journal*, 19:1929–1934.

Collins FS, Guttmacher AE (2001). Genetics moves into the medical mainstream. *Journal of the American Medical Association*, 286:2322–2324.

Doerge RW (2002). Mapping and analysis of quantitative trait loci in experimental populations. *Nature Reviews Genetics*, 3:42–52.

Gardener R (2001). Stem cell therapy – problems and prospects. *Science and Public Affairs* (Aug 2001):5.

Guerinot ML (2000). The green revolution strikes gold. *Science*, 287:241–243.

Hashmi S, Tawe W, Lustigman S (2001). *Caenorhabditis elegans* and the study of gene function in parasites. *Trends in Parasitology*, 17:387–393.

Interagency Working Group on Microbial Genomics (2001). *The microbe project report*. US National Science and Technology Council, Committee on Science, Subcommittee on Biotechnology (Accessed at http://www.ostp.gov/html/microbial/pdf_files/aboutus.pdf Jan 16, 2002)

Khoury MJ, Burke W, Thompson EJ (eds) (2000). *Genetics and Public Health in the 21st Century*. Oxford, Oxford University Press.

Reich DE, Cargill M, Bolk S, Ireland J, Sabeti PC, Richter DJ, et al. (2001). Linkage disequilbrium in the human genome. *Nature*, 411:199–204.

Relman DA, Falkow S (2001). The meaning and impact of the human genome sequence for microbiology. *Trends in Microbiology*, 9:206–208.

Schultze JL, Vonderheide RH (2001). From cancer genomics to cancer immunotherapy: toward second generation tumor antigens. *Trends in Immunology*, 22:516–523.

Subramanian G, Adams MD, Venter JC, Broder S (2001). Implications of the human genome for understanding human biology and medicine. *Journal of the American Medical Association*, 286:2296–2307.

Williamson, B (2001). Our human genome – how can it serve us well. *Bulletin of the World Health Organization*, 79:1005.

SECTION 4

References

Altmuller J, Palmer LJ, Fischer G, Scherb H, Wjst M (2001). Genomewide scans of complex human diseases: true linkage is hard to find. *American Journal of Human Genetics*, 69:936–950.

Burn J, Duff G, Holtzman NA (2001). Three views of genetics: the enthusiast, the visionary, and the sceptic. *British Medical Journal*, 322:1016.

Commission on Macroeconomics and Health (2001). *Macroeconomics and Health: Investing in Health for Economic Development*. Geneva, WHO

Harris E, Tanner M (2000). Health technology transfer. *British Medical Journal*, 321:817–820.

Roos DS (2001). Bioinformatics – trying to swim in a sea of data. *Science*, 291:1260–1261.

Weatherall DJ (1999). From genotype to phenotype: genetics and medical practice in the new millennium. *Philosophical Transactions of the Royal Society of London Series B*, 354:1995–2010.

WHO (1994). *Guidelines for the Control of Haemoglobin Disorders. Reports of the VIth Annual Meeting of the WHO Working Group on Haemoglobinopathies.* Geneva, World Health Organization. (Accessed at http://whqlibdoc.who.int/hq/1994/WHO_HDP_HB_GL_94.1.pdf Jan 16, 2002)

Widdus R (2001). Public-private partnerships for health: their main targets, their diversity, and their future directions. *Bulletin of the World Health Organization*, 79:713–720.

Wilkie AOM (2001). Genetic predictions:what are the limits? *Stud. Hist. Phil. Biol. Biomed. Sci.*, 32:619–633.

Further Reading

Childs B, Valle D (2000). Genetics, Biology and Disease. *Annual Review of Genomics and Human Genetics*, 1:1–19.

Holtzman NA (2001). Putting the search for genes in perspective. *International Journal of Health Services* 31:445–461.

Holtzman NA, Marteau TM (2000). Will genetics revolutionize medicine? *New England Journal of Medicine* 343:141–144.

Hoover RN (2000). Cancer – nature, nurture or both. *New England Journal of Medicine*, 343:135–136.

Michaud CM, Murray CJL, Bloom BR (2001). Burden of disease – implications for future research. *Journal of American Medical Association*, 285:535–539.

Weatherall DJ (2000). Internal Medicine in the 21st Century – Introduction. *Journal of Internal Medicine*, 247:3–5.

SECTION 5

References

Alberti G (2001). Noncommunicable diseases: tomorrow's pandemics. *Bulletin of the World Health Organization*, 79:907.

Cooke GS, Hill AVS (2001). Genetics of susceptibility to human infectious disease. *Nature Reviews Genetics*, 2:967–977.

de Silva S, Fisher CA, Premawardhena A, Lamabadusuriya SP, Peto TEA, Perera G, et al. (2000). Thalassemia in Sri Lanka: implications for the future health burden of Asian populations. *The Lancet*, 355:786–791.

Djimdé A, Doumbo OK, Steketee RW, Plowe CV (2001). Application of a molecular marker for surveillance of chloroquine-resistant falciparum malaria *The Lancet*, 358:890–891.

Harris E, Lopez M, Arevalo J, Bellatin J, Belli A, Moran J, et al. (1993). Short courses on DNA detection and amplification in Central and South America: The democratization of molecular biology. *Biochemical Education*, 21:16–22.

Harris E, Tanner M. (2000). Health technology transfer. *British Medical Journal*, 321:817–820.

Hassan MHA (2001). Can science save Africa? *Science*, 292:1609.

Schaeffeler E, Eichelbaum M, Brinkmann U, Penger A, Asante-Poku S, Zanger UM, et al. (2001). Frequency of C3435T polymorphism of MDR1 gene in African people. *The Lancet*, 358:383–384.

Unwin N, Setel P, Rashid S, Mugusi F, Mbanya JC, Kitange H, et al. (2001). Noncommunicable diseases in sub-Saharan Africa: where do they feature in the health research agenda. *Bulletin of the World Health Organization*, 79:947–953.

Weatherall DJ, Clegg JB (2001). Inherited haemoglobin disorders: an increasing global health problem. *Bulletin of the World Health Organization*, 79:704–712.

WHO (1997). Alwan A (ed). *Community control of genetic and congenital disorders*. EMRO Technical Publications, Series 24. Alexandria, WHO (EMRO). (Accessed at http://www.emro.who.int/Publications/EMRO%20PUB-TPS-GEN.HTM Jan 16, 2002)

WHO (2000). *Primary health care approaches for prevention and control of congenital and genetic disorders*. (document WHO/HGN/WG/00.1). (Accessed at http://www.who.int/ncd/hgn/hcprevention.htm Jan 16, 2002)

Zimmet P, Alberti KGMM, Shaw J (2001). Global and societal implications of the diabetes epidemic. *Nature*, 414:782–787.

Further Reading

Bloom BR, Trach DD (2001). Genetics and developing countries. *British Medical Journal*, 322:1006–1007.

Cassell GH, Mekalanos J (2001). Development of antimicrobial agents in the era of new and reemerging infectious diseases and increasing antibiotic resistance. *Journal of the American Medical Association*, 285:601–605.

Catteruccia F, Nolan T, Loukeris TG, Blass C, Savakis C, Kafatos FC, et al. (2000). Stable germline transformation of the malaria mosquito *Anopheles stephensi*. *Nature*, 405:959–962.

Enserink M (2001). Two new steps towards a "better mosquito." *Science*, 293:2370–2371.

Jasinskiene N, Coates CJ, Benedict MQ, Cornel AJ, Rafferty CS, James AA, et al. (1998). Stable transformation of the yellow fever mosquito, *Aedes aegypti*, with the Hermes element from the housefly. *Proceedings of the National Academy of Sciences USA*, 95:3743–3747.

Letvin NL, Bloom BR, Hoffman SL (2001). Prospects for vaccines to protect against AIDS, tuberculosis and malaria. *Journal of the American Medical Association*, 285:606–611.

Martinson JL, Chapman NH, Rees DC, Liu.YT, Clegg JB (1997). Global distribution of the CCR5 gene 32-basepair deletion. *Nature Genetics* 16:100–102.

Orme IM, McMurray DN, Belisle JT (2001). Tuberculosis vaccine development: recent progress. *Trends in Microbiology*, 9:115–118.

Rathod PK, Ganesan K, Hayward RE, Bozdech Z, DeRisi JL (2002). DNA microarrays for malaria. *Trends in Parasitology*, 18:39–45.

Seder RA, Hill AVS (2000). Vaccines against intracellular infections requiring cellular immunity. *Nature*, 406:793–798.

Simpson AJG (2001). Genome sequencing networks. *Nature Reviews Genetics*, 2:979–983

Taylor LH, Latham SM, Woolhouse ME (2001). Risk factors for human disease emergence. *Philosophical Transactions of the Royal Society of London Series B*, 356:983–989.

Zagury D, Burny A, Gallo RC (2001). Toward a new generation of vaccines: the anti-cytokine therapeutic vaccines. *Proceedings of the National Academy of Sciences USA*, 98:8024–8029.

SECTION 6

References

Chadwick R, Berg K (2001). Solidarity and equity: new ethical frameworks for genetic data bases. *Nature Reviews Genetics*, 2:318–321.

Fraser CM, Dando MR (2001). Genomics and future biological weapons: the need for preventive action by the biomedical community. *Nature Genetics*, 29:253–256.

Fukuyama F (2002). Our Posthuman Future: Consequences of the Biotechnology Revolution. New York, Farrar, Strauss and Giroux.

Gasson M, Burke D (2001): Scientific perspectives on regulating the safety of genetically modified foods. *Nature Reviews Genetics*, 2:217–222.

Malakoff D, Enserink M (2001). New law may force labs to screen workers. *Science*, 294:971–973.

Modell B, Khan M, Darlison M, King A, Layton M, Old J, et al. (2001). A national register for surveillance of inherited disorders: beta thalassaemia in the United Kingdom. *Bulletin of the World Health Organization*, 79:1006–1013.

Neel JV (2000). Some ethical issues at the population level raised by 'soft' eugenics, euphenics, and isogenics. *Human Hereditary*, 50:14–21.

Reilly P (2001). Legal and public policy issues in DNA forensics. *Nature Reviews Genetics*, 2:313–317.

Robertson JA (2001). Human embryonic stem cell research: ethical and legal issues. *Nature Reviews Genetics*, 2:74–78.

Further Reading

Fears R, Poste G (1999). Building population genetics resources using the UK NHS. *Science*, 284:267–268.

Meselson M (2000). Averting the hostile exploitation of biotechnology. *CBW Conventions Bulletin*, 48:16–19

UK Royal Society (2001). *The use of genetically modified animals*. London, The Royal Society (Accessed at http://www.royalsoc.ac.uk/policy/index.html Jan 16, 2002)

SECTION 7

References

Barton J (2001). Research tool patents – issues for developing world health. *Bulletin of the World Health Organization* (in press).

Bear JC (2001). What is a person's DNA worth? Fair compensation for DNA access. Paper presented at the 10th *International Congress of Human Genetics*, Vienna, May. (Accessed at http://www.mannvernd.is/english/articles/jb_fair_compensation.html Dec 10, 2001)

Bobrow M, Thomas S (2001). Patents in a genetic age. *Nature*, 409:763–764.

Buse K, Waxman A (2001). Public–private health partnerships: a strategy for WHO. *Bulletin of the World Health Organization*, 79:748–754.

Cherry M (2001). Health priorities gain patent reprieve for developing countries. *Nature*, 414:385

Commission on Macroeconomics and Health (2001). *Macroeconomics and Health: Investing in Health for Economic Development*. Geneva, WHO

Convention on Biological Diversity (CBD). (Accessed at http://www.biodiv.org Dec 10, 2001)

Cook-Deegan R, Chan C, Johnson A (2000). *World survey of funding for genomics research, final report*. Prepared for the Global Forum for Health Research and the WHO. (Accessed at http://www.stanford.edu/class/siw198q/websites/genomics/finalrpt.htm Jan 16, 2002)

Dutfield G (2001). *The Andean Pact Common System on Access to Genetic Resources: A commentary*. Paper posted at website of Working Group on Traditional Resource Rights, Oxford Centre for Environment, Ethics and Society: (Accessed at http://users.ox.ac.uk/~wgtrr/andpacomm.htm Jan 16, 2002)

Global Forum for Health Research (2000). *The 10/90 Report on Health Research 2000*. Geneva, Global Forum for Health Research.

Global Health Forum I (2000). *Creating Global Markets for Neglected Drugs and Vaccines: A Challenge for Public-Private Partnerships*. Consensus statement of the Global Health Forum I, 18–21 February 2000.(Accessed at http://www.epibiostat.ucsf.edu/igh/programs/GlobalForumI.pdf Jan 16, 2002)

HUGO (2000). *Statement on Patenting of DNA Sequences.* (Accessed at http://www.hugo-international.org/hugo/patent2000.html Dec 10, 2001)

Lucas A (2000). *Public-private partnerships: Illustrative Examples.* Extracts from a paper presented at a workshop on public-private partnerships in public health, Massachusetts, USA, 7–8 April, 2000. (Accessed at http://www.who.int/tdr Jan 16, 2002)

Millenium Africa Recovery Plan. (Accessed at http://www.africainitiative.org/home.asp Dec 10, 2001)

Pecoul B, Chirac P, Trouiller P, Pinel J (1999). Access to essential drugs in poor countries: A lost battle? *Journal of the American Medical Association,* 281:361–367.

Service RF. (2001). Gene and protein patents get ready to go head to head. *Science,* 294:2082–2083.

Sykes R (2000). *New Medicines, the Practice of Medicine and Public Policy.* London, The Stationery Office.

UNDP (2001). *Human Development Report 2001 — Making New Technologies Work for Human Development.* New York, Oxford University Press for the United Nations Development Program.

UNESCO, IBC (2001). *The International Symposium of Ethics, Intellectual Property and Genomics — Final Report.* (Accessed at http://www.unesco.org/ibc/ Dec 10, 2001).

United Kingdom House of Lords Select Committee on Science and Technology (2001). *Human Genetic Databases: Challenges and Opportunities.* Fourth Report. (Accessed at http://www.parliament.the-stationery-office.co.uk/pa/ld200001/ldselect/ldsctech/57/5701.htm Jan 16, 2002)

Wasi P (2001). *Genomics and health: South East Asian perspectives.* Paper presented at the WHO Multi-regional Consultative Meeting on Genomics and Health, Thailand, 23–25 July 2001.

WHO Programme of Nutrition (1997). *WHO Global Database on Child Growth and Malnutrition.* Geneva, World Health Organization. (document WHO/NUT/97.4) (Accessed at http://www.who.int/nutgrowthdb/ Jan 16, 2002)

WHO (1999). *The World Health Report 1999 — Making a Difference in People's Lives: Achievements and Challenges.* Geneva, World Health Organization.

WHO and WTO Secretariats (2001). *Workshop on Differential Pricing and Financing of Essential Drugs, Executive Summary of Report,* Hosbjor, Norway. (Accessed at http://www.who.int/medicines/library/edm_general/who-wto-hosbjor/hosbjorexe-eng.pdf Jan 16, 2002)

Widdus R (2001). Public–private partnerships for health: their main targets, their diversity, and their future directions. *Bulletin of the World Health Organization,* 79:713–720.

Williamson AR (2001). Gene patents: socially acceptable monopolies or an unnecessary hindrance to research? *Trends in Genetics,* 17:670–673.

World Trade Organization (2001). *Declaration on the TRIPS Agreement and Public Health*.Ministerial Conference, Fourth Session, Doha 9–14 November 2001, adopted on 14 November 2001. (document WT/MIN(01)/DEC/2). (Accessed at http://docsonline.wto.org/gen_home.asp Jan 16, 2002)

Further Reading

Amir Attaran, Gillespie-White L (2001). Do patents for antiretroviral drugs constrain access to AIDS Treatment in Africa? *Journal of the American Medical Association*, 286:1886–1892.

Burgess MM (2001). Beyond consent: ethical and social issues in genetic testing. *Nature Reviews Genetics*, 2:147–151.

Caulfield T, Gold ER, Cho MK (2000). Patenting human genetic material: refocusing the debate. *Nature Reviews Genetics*, 1:227–231.

Chee HL, El-Hamamsy L, Fleming J, Fujiki N, Keyeux G, Knoppers BM et al. (1996). Bioethics and human population genetics research in *Proceedings of the Third Session of the IBC of UNESCO, 1995, Volume I*. Paris, UNESCO, 39 –64.

Correa CM (2001). Health and intellectual property rights. *Bulletin of the World Health Organization*, 79:381.

Global Health Forum II (2000). *Intellectual Property Rights and Global Health: Challenges for Access and Research and Development*. Global Health Forum II, 7–9 December 2000. (Accessed at http://www.epibiostat.ucsf.edu/igh/programs/GlobalForumII.pdf Jan 16, 2002)

Rabino I (2001). How human geneticists in US view commercialization of the Human Genome Project. *Nature Genetics*, 29:15–16.

Rifkin J (1999). *The Biotech Century: Harnessing the Gene and Remaking the World*. New York, Penguin Putman Inc.

UNESCO (2000). *Intellectual Property in the Field on the Human Genome – Preliminary Analysis of Available Documents*. (Accessed at http://www.unesco.org/ethics/en/Documents/Background/intprop_en.rtf Dec 10, 2001)

Weatherall DJ (1997). Medical research in the next millennium: the case for a partnership between the richer countries and the developing world. *RSA Journal* (July):56–64.

Widdus R (2001). Public-private partnerships for health: their main targets, their diversity, and their future directions. *Bulletin of the World Health Organization*, 79:713–720.

SECTION 8

References

Davis D (2001) Genetic Dilemmas: Reproductive Technology, Parental Choices, and Children's Futures. London, Routledge Publishers.

Faden RR, Beauchamp TL (1986) A History and Theory of Informed Consent. New York, Oxford University Press.

Gulcher JR, Stefansson K (2000) The Icelandic Healthcare Database and Informed Consent. New England Journal of Medicine, 342:1827–30.

Nuffield Council on Bioethics (1993) Genetic Screening: Ethical Issues. London, Nuffield Council on Bioethics. (Accessed at http://www.nuffieldbioethics.org/filelibrary/pdf/genetic_screening.pdf Jan 16, 2002)

Parens E (ed) (1998) Enhancing Human Traits: Ethical and Social Implications. Washington DC, Georgetown University Press.

Parens E, Asch A (eds) (2000) Prenatal Testing and Disability Rights. Washington DC, Georgetown University Press.

Paul D (1995) Controlling Human Heredity, 1865 to the Present. Atlantic Highlands NJ, Humanities Press.

Robertson JA (2001). Human embryonic stem cell research: ethical and legal issues. Nature Reviews Genetics, 2:74–77.

Rothenberg KH, Thomson EJ (eds) (1994) Women and Prenatal Testing: Facing the Challenges of Genetic Technology. Columbus, Ohio State University Press.

Rothstein MA (ed) (1997) Genetic Secrets: Protecting Privacy and Confidentiality in the Genetic Era. New Haven CT, Yale University Press.

Vogelstein B, Alberts B, Shine K (2002). Please don't call it cloning!. *Science*, 295:1237.

Further Reading

Annas G, Elias S (eds) (1992) *Gene Mapping: Using Law and Ethics as Guides*. New York, Oxford University Press.

Buchanan AE, Brock DW, Daniels N, Wikler D (2000) *From Chance to Choice: Genetics and Justice*. Cambridge, Cambridge University Press.

Daar AS, Mattei JF (1999): Medical Genetics and Biotechnology: Implications for Public Health. Annex 1 in *Ethical Issues in Genetics, Cloning and Biotechnology: possible future directions for WHO*. Report of an informal con sultation. Geneva, World Health Organization. (document WHO/EIP/GPE/00.1)

Disabled Peoples International—Europe (2001). *Position Statement on Bioethics and Human Rights*. (Accessed at http://www.dpieurope.org/htm/bioethics/dpsngfullre- port.htm January 30, 2002)

Andrews LB, Fullarton JE, Holtzman NA, Motulsky AG (eds) (1994) *Assessing Genetic Risks: Implications for Health and Social Policy*. Washington DC, National Academy Press.

Lauritzen P (ed) (2001) *Cloning and the Future of Human Embryo Research*. Oxford, Oxford University Press.

Singer PA, Daar AS (2001). Harnessing genomics and biotechnology to improve global health equity. *Science*, 294:87 89.

UNESCO (1997) *Universal Declaration on the Human Genome and Human Rights*. Paris, United Nations Educational, Scientific and Cultural Organization. (Accessed at http://www.unesco.org/ibc/en/genome/ Jan 16, 2002)

UNESCO (2001) *Report of the IBC on Solidarity and International Co-operation between Developed and Developing Countries Concerning the Human Genome*. Paris, United Nations Educational, Scientific and Cultural Organization.

Walters L, Palmer JG (1997) *The Ethics of Human Gene Therapy*. New York, Oxford University Press.

Weir RF, Lawrence SC, Fales E (eds) (1994) *Genes and Human Self-Knowledge: Historical and Philosophical Reflections on Modern Genetics*. Iowa City, University of Iowa Press.

WHO (1998) *Proposed International Guidelines on Ethical Issues in Medical Genetics and Genetic Services*. Report of a WHO Meeting on Ethical Issues in Medical Genetics. Geneva, World Health Organization. (document WHO/HGN/GL/ETH/98.1)

WHO (1999) *Cloning in Human Health* – Report by the Secretariat. Geneva, World Health Organization. (Accessed at http://www.who.int/gb/EB_WHA/PDF/WHA52/ew12.pdf Jan 16, 2002)

SECTION 9

References

Cao A, Rosatelli MC (1993). Screening and prenatal diagnosis of haemoglobinopathies. *Baillieres Clinical Haematology*, 6:263–286.

Macer D, Bezar H, Harman N, Kamada H, Macer NY (1997). Attitudes to Biotechnology in Japan and New Zealand in 1997, with International Comparisons. *Eubios Journal of Asian and International Bioethics*, 7:137–151.

National Center for Genome Resources, USA (1998). *National Attitudes of Public and Stakeholder Attitudes and Awareness of Genetic Issues* (Accessed at http://www.ncgr.org Jan 16, 2002)

Nuffield Council on Bioethics (1993). Genetic screening and public policy. In *Genetic Screening Ethical Issues*. London, Nuffield Council on Bioethics, 75–81.

Office of Science and Technology (2000). *Science and the Public. A review of science and communication and public attitudes to science in Britain*. (Accessed at http://www.dti.gov.uk/ost/aboutost/index.htm Jan 16, 2002)

Richmond MH, Mattison N, Williams P. (1999). *Human Genomics. Prospects for Health Care and Public Policy*. London, Pharmaceutical Partners for Better Health Care.

Scriver CR, Bardanis M, Cartier L, Clow CL, Lancaster GA, Ostrowsky JT (1984). β-thalassemia disease prevention: genetic medicine applied. *American Journal of Human Genetics*, 36:1024–1038.

Wellcome Trust (1998). *Public perspectives on human cloning.* Medicine and Society Programme, The Wellcome Trust, London. (Accessed at http://www.wellcome.ac.uk/en/images/cloning_report_slimversion_2816.pdf Jan 16, 2002)

Further Reading

Condit C (2001). What is "public opinion" about genetics?. *Nature Reviews Genetics,* 2:811–815.

Durant J, Bauer MW, Gaskel G (eds) (1998). *Biotechnology in the Public Sphere: A European Sourcebook.* London, Science Museum.

Durant J, Hansen A, Bauer M (1994). Public understanding of the new genetics. In Marteau R, Richards M (eds.) *The Troubled Helix: social and psychological implications of the new human genetics.* Cambridge, Cambridge University Press 235–248.

National Reference Center for Bioethics Literature (2000) Scope Note 22: *Genetic Testing and Genetic Screening.* (Accessed at http://www.georgetown.edu/research/nrcbl/scopenotes/sn22.htm Jan 20, 2002)

Nelkin, D (2001). Molecular metaphors: the gene in popular discourse. *Nature Reviews Genetics,* 2:555–559.

Neuberger J (2000). The educated patient: new challenges for the medical profession. *Journal of Internal Medicine,* 247:6–10.

Office of Science and Technology and the Wellcome Trust (2000). *Science and the Public – a review of science communication and public attitudes to science in Britain.* London, Office of Science and Technology and the Wellcome Trust.(Accessed at http://www.wellcome.ac.uk/en/images/sciencepublic_3391.pdf Jan 18, 2002)

Paabo S (2001). The human genome and our view of ourselves. *Science,* 291:1219–1220.

Schiele B, Amyot M, Benoit C (eds)(1994). *When Science Becomes Culture: World Survey of Scientific Culture.* Quebec, University of Ottawa Press.

Wynne B (2000). Retrieving a human agenda for science. *RSA Journal,* 2(4): 4–6

Figure 2.5 MICROARRAY (DNA CHIP) TECHNOLOGY *(see page 34)*

In this experiment human DNA has been incorporated into a series of microchips. To establish which genes are activated when a particular cell line is transformed by Epstein-Barr (EB) virus, total RNA was extracted from the transformed cells and converted to complementary DNA (cDNA); in this process the cDNA was labeled with a fluorescent dye (Cy3). The labelled cDNA was then applied to the chip. The colour signals vary according to the activity of the genes in the cell line. Each chip shows a doublet in one corner, called Cy3 landing lights, which are simply to orientate the position of the genes on the chip.

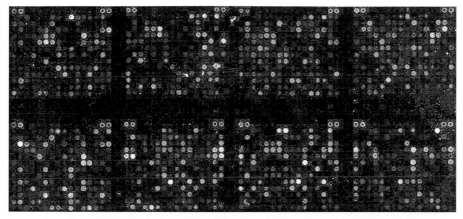

(Figure supplied by the courtesy of AT Merryweather-Clarke, C Langford, D Vetrie and KJH Robson, Weatherall Institute of Molecular Medicine, Oxford, United Kingdom)

Figure 3.3 MULTICOLOUR FLUORESCENT *in situ* HYBRIDISATION (FISH)
ANALYSIS OF CHROMASOMES *(see page 59)*

The upper figure shows a normal human male set of chromosomes. Each chromosome is
identified by a different combination of fluorescent dyes attached to specific DNA fragments which bind to particular human chromosomes. This method allows the detection of
inter-chromosomal rearrangements and other chromosomal abnormalities. Each chromosome can be identified by its particular colour. The lower figure shows the chromosomes
of a gibbon, which has 38 chromosomes. These have been analysed using a human FISH
probe. The multicoloured chromosomes show the remarkable interchromosomal
rearrangements which have occurred during the divergence of humans and gibbons over
14 million years.

(Figure kindly supplied by Dr. Willem Rens and Professor Malcolm Ferguson-Smith).

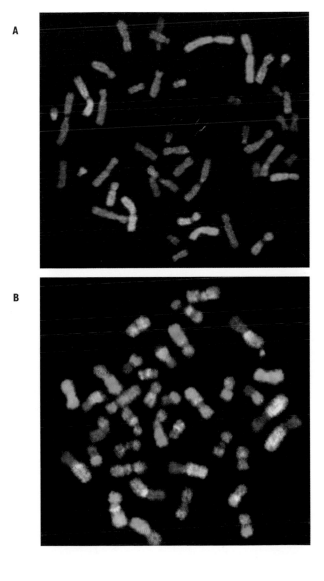